THE MYSTERY OF THE EYE
AND THE SHADOW OF BLINDNESS

Blindness is commonly considered to be a physical condition with negative consequences for those affected. Most research and treatment begin with the assumption that blind persons require adjustment and training to cope with their distorted view of reality. For Rod Michalko, blindness offers a legitimate way of being and a teaching tool – one that presents a unique perspective on aspects of the world that the sighted never experience and that the disciplines of ophthalmology and rehabilitation never consider.

This book explores matters of choice and personal fulfilment in the context of blindness. Ophthalmology and rehabilitation use sheer necessity as their guiding principle, but the blind person must grapple with the question of what kind of blind person he or she chooses to be. The story of blindness is retold in the life of every blind person and whenever blindness is thought about, spoken of, or acted upon. Michalko immerses himself in this multiplicity of narration, weaving his own experience of blindness through it, using it as an occasion to think about life, our decisions, our choices, including how we choose to understand each other, and the ways we choose to live collectively in the human community. He wants readers to consider what can be produced by thinking of blindness as an essential part of being.

This is an important book for anyone who has personal or professional contact with any community of disabled persons, particularly the blind, as well as anyone who simply wants to better understand what it means to be human.

ROD MICHALKO is Adjunct Professor of Sociology in the Department of Sociology and Anthropology at Saint Francis Xavier University. Until recently he was a senior trainer at the Management Board Secretariat for the Ontario government.

ROD MICHALKO

The Mystery of the Eye
and the Shadow of Blindness

UNIVERSITY OF TORONTO PRESS
Toronto Buffalo London

© University of Toronto Press Incorporated 1998
Toronto Buffalo London
Printed in Canada

ISBN 0-8020-4250-3 (cloth)
ISBN 0-8020-8093-6 (paper)

Printed on acid-free paper

Canadian Cataloguing in Publication Data

Michalko, Rodney Leonard, 1946–
  The mystery of the eye and the shadow of blindness

  Includes bibliographical references and index.
  ISBN 0-8020-4250-3 (bound)   ISBN 0-8020-8093-6 (pbk.)

  1. Blindness – Social aspects.   I. Title.

  HV1593.M53 1998   362.4′1   C97-931455-0

University of Toronto Press acknowledges the financial assistance to its
publishing program of the Canada Council for the Arts and the
Ontario Arts Council.

For Tanya

Contents

Acknowledgments

This book took shape quite innocently. I began by organizing my thoughts about blindness in accordance with how I experienced it. This developed into a consideration of how others experience their blindness as well as how our society and its institutions conceive of blindness. This work was my way of attempting to come to an understanding of my own blindness.

I showed this work to Heather Berkeley, who encouraged me to seek out a publisher; I am thus indebted to Heather for steering me onto the road of publication. This road led me to University of Toronto Press, and I am especially indebted to Virgil Duff, Executive Editor, who worked very patiently with me in bringing this work to fruition. Ken Lewis copy-edited the manuscript with a sensitivity that maintained and even enhanced the integrity of my work. I used a Dictaphone to generate the first draft of this book, and I am indebted to Gord Taylor, who spent countless hours transcribing my dictation. I am also indebted to Kate Anderson, Mark Lede, and Tara Milbrandt for the care and patience they brought to the proofreading of this work. And I am especially grateful for the creative way in which they indexed it.

I owe much to the scores of blind persons I have come to know over the years. Many of them told me their stories of blindness, and we had many hours of discussion about the meaning of blindness and how our society treats blind persons. I am also indebted to the parents of blind children who spoke freely with me of their experiences. Many professionals in the fields of ophthalmology, rehabilitation, and education spoke with me about blindness. Without these various experiences with blindness, this book would not have been written.

One of the most interesting contributors to this book is my god-daughter, Beth. At the time of her birth, I had approximately 10 per cent of 'normal' vision. As Beth grew, so did my blindness. She experienced several different godfathers in relation to my diminishing sight. Beth tried her best to understand my ever-changing eyesight. At times she was surprised, at other times compassionate, and at still other times she responded with humour. She was always curious. Beth played with my blindness and found that she could easily trick me. For example, when we were in a cafe, she would offer to help me find the washroom and lead me right to the door marked 'Women.' Beth also played at being blind, using my white cane as though it was, as she put it at age six, 'the funnest thing.' Beth mirrored my own responses to my blindness. I learned much from her in regard to the development of an imaginative relation to blindness.

Finally, I am most grateful to my partner in life, Dr Tanya Titchkosky. Tanya lived my blindness with me for the past eight years. During the last four years, my sight diminished to almost nothing. This had some unexpected consequences for my life. The most surprising of them was that the more sight I lost, the more Tanya enjoyed my blindness. Enjoyment was a reaction to blindness which I had never experienced before. This made me consider the possibility of enjoying blindness and thus enjoying life as a blind person. Tanya has lived every sentence of this book with me, and she continues to enjoy blindness. She has taught me to allow my blindness to become a teacher.

THE MYSTERY OF THE EYE
AND THE SHADOW OF BLINDNESS

1

Introduction

This book is a culmination of many things. First, and I think most important, it represents the way in which I have come to think about my own experience as a blind person. Experiencing blindness, however, is not in any way synonymous with knowledge. The adage that 'experience is the best teacher' is true, but it is only true when experience is *allowed* to teach. And, it is only recently that I have allowed my blindness to assume the role of teacher. This means that my experience of being blind is something that can be thought about, and this book is an attempt to represent those thoughts and to represent the knowledge that I have gained through my experience.

Second, this book represents thoughts about my experience with the many blind persons I have come to know over the years. Some of them have become very close friends, others are acquaintances, and still others are people whom I do not like. Each blind person chooses to exemplify and to live his or her blindness in a particular way. This book attempts to capture the value of these various examples of living the life of blindness.

Third, this book represents thoughts about my professional work with blind persons. I spent part of my life as a counsellor working with blind children, blind adolescents, their parents, their educators, and so on. This experience, and the idea that professional intervention is a taken-for-granted necessity in the life of blind persons, has inspired me to think about the ways our society is organized such that it conceives of blind persons as requiring professional help and how it proceeds to organize this help. What counts as 'help' has taught me more about our society than it has about blindness. It has taught me what our society thinks blindness is and how our society tells blind persons what they are, how to act, and how to conceive of themselves.

Fourth, this book represents the culmination of many years of research on blindness. This research began when I decided to make blindness a topic for both my M.A. and Ph.D. studies. I have since conducted many research projects in relation to blindness. The fact that blindness is treated as a legitimate topic for academic research has inspired me to think about the ways in which we conceive of not seeing, or not seeing well, as topical within the world of academia. This has led me to consider how the various academic disciplines, from ophthalmology to psychology, have subjected blindness as something worthy of their investigations.

Finally, much of what I have learned about blindness has come from people who are not blind. These people, my friends, people with whom I live and whom I love, relate to me, in part, as someone who is blind. The way they relate to me tells me not only something about myself but also something about their conception of blindness. Their relation to me is a relation that takes into account the fact that I am blind. I have spent most of my life living with the idea that I am a person first and blind second. These people have taught me that my blindness is part of who I am and that I am not a person who 'happens to be blind' but, instead, that I am a 'blind person.' They have taught me that blindness has influenced my life and that I would be a different person were I not blind.

This book is not about me but is about blindness itself. In the final analysis, the culmination of all my experiences has been that they have led me to that place from which I can ask the question What is blindness?

This book represents my attempt to think about blindness. It is not a 'how to do it' book. It is not a book that will tell you how to cope with your blindness or how to cope with the blindness of others. It is a book that will invite you to embrace blindness as an occasion to think about life, our choices, our decisions, how we choose to understand each other, and the ways in which we choose to live collectively in the human community. It is a book that elevates blindness to the position of something which provokes thought. This book represents my attempt to raise blindness out of the quagmire of sheer necessity into the horizon of possibilities that comes with the luxury produced when blindness is thought of as an essential part of being.

The first step in this attempt is to treat blindness as a story. It has something to tell us about the human community and about what we value as individuals and as a collective. There are many tellers of the story of blindness, and their voices are heard in activities such as diagnosis, medicine, rehabilitation, and so on. I will give voice to these various tellers of the story throughout the chapters of this book.

However, the two most important voices in the story of blindness are those of sightedness and blindness. It is the conversation between the two, and how they interact with one another in the world, that shows us the meaning of both. Thus, I begin in chapter 2 with two fictional accounts of blindness: the first depicts a sighted person stumbling into a country which is inhabited only by blind persons; the second depicts a conversation between a blind and a sighted person in a world largely inhabited by people who see. These narratives frame both blindness and sightedness as stories which unfold in the interaction they have with one another. In the first story, the sighted character, Nunez, represents sight living in the *Country of the Blind* (H.G. Wells, 1927). In the second, Jenny, a blind woman, represents blindness living in the 'Country of the Sighted.' These characters appear throughout the book as guides to the telling of the story of blindness. With these stories as a springboard, I devote the rest of chapter 2 to raising the question What is blindness?

Chapter 3 is devoted to a discussion of the 'discovery of blindness.' Blindness is present to all of us by virtue of its opposite – sight. Nevertheless, this needs to be discovered. A discovery of blindness also takes place when an individual loses her or his sight or is born without it. Blindness is not obvious. I make use of stories that I have collected from many blind persons and from parents of blind children as a way to show how blindness is discovered and how it becomes obvious.

Blindness is also diagnosed. Diagnosis relies upon common sense in that it assumes what normal seeing life 'looks like.' 'Normal seeing' provides the background against which an instance of blindness can be discovered. We know we are blind and we know when others are blind when the appearance of normal seeing disappears. Diagnosis enters the story of blindness at this point. It explains the discovery of blindness by attributing a medical cause to it as well as giving it a prognosis. Diagnosis is the final arbiter: if the prognosis is positive, blindness is prevented; if negative, another blind person enters the world.

In chapter 4 I will address blindness from the point of view of the 'problem of knowledge.' Blindness is often understood as a problem of knowing insofar as knowledge is understood as springing from sense perception. If we possess our senses in natural working order, we possess knowledge. A glance at any current introductory psychology text shows the modern understanding that most of what we know comes through our senses, and it shows that most of *that knowing* comes through our sense of sight. This conception of knowledge and knowing sets up an obvious connection: the less we see, the less we know. This connection is what the work of rehabilitation begins and ends with.

I address this issue by examining rehabilitation and educational main-streaming programs. These programs evoke various techniques for solving the problem of blindness understood as the problem of knowledge. Their essential aim is to provide blind persons with skills which will allow them to adapt to a sighted world. Thus, 'fitting in' society is what these programs have in mind for blind persons. They want blind persons to be like everyone else – just persons. Person is first, blindness is second. Persons who *happen* to be blind are what these programs hope to release into the world.

Rehabilitation programs conceive of blindness as a mere shadow of sight. Their goal is to make blind persons appear as ordinary as possible. Blind persons are just like everyone else and, with the right techniques, they can do the things that everyone else does. Adolescents have the same thing in mind. Each teenager wants to be like every other teenager. Teenagers want to walk in the same way, talk in the same way, dress in the same way, and so on. Rehabilitation wants this for blind persons in that it wants blind persons to do the ordinary things that ordinary people do. By stressing ordinary personhood, rehabilitation hopes to diminish the extraordinariness of blindness.

We all know that adolescence is a time of turbulence. It is also a temporary time. This is a time when we want to be like everyone else; collective life overrides individual life. In chapter 5 I will develop the theme of adolescence in relation to blindness that I raised in chapter 4. I will show how a blind adolescent succumbs to the temptation of passing as sighted, as acting as if he or she can see. This is the story of my adolescence. This is what I did. With my life as the example, I will demonstrate how blind persons are tempted to act in as ordinary a way as possible. Being average and normal is the aim of this life; it is also the aim of rehabilitation. It is no different from adolescence in this regard. Both hold out the promise of the average life.

Chapter 6 will address the need for developing a mature relation to blindness. To this point, the voices in the story of blindness have spoken of it as a lack and as 'something missing.' As such, their commitment was to alleviating this lack. They were not interested in learning anything from it. This chapter will show that blindness has much to teach us. It can teach us that sight is not so clearly known as ophthalmology and rehabilitation make it out to be. There is a mystery in eyesight which blindness can show us. Blindness does not have to be a mere shadow of sight. It can be as mysterious as the eye. Blindness can teach us about the essential mystery of human life and the need to keep this mystery alive. It can teach us that the question What is blindness?

is never answered once and for all. Each answer is asking the question once again and for the first time. Blindness is not ordinary. It provides *everyone* with the occasion to think about what is important and reminds *everyone* that a thoughtful life is more valuable than an ordinary one.

We now have a story of blindness. This book, with all of its chapters, takes blindness from discovery to maturity. It makes use of many examples. These examples come from the 'real lives' of blind persons, of professionals of various kinds, and of those who are intimately connected with blind persons; they show what it means to be blind and how to live with that condition. This book itself is an example. It not only exemplifies the need to understand blindness as a condition that must be coped with, but also it exemplifies the need to treat blindness, or any condition, as an occasion to think about what is important, what is worthwhile, and what is valuable.

I conclude this book in the same way I began it – with a story. The story depicts a conversation between a blind person and a sighted person. They are discussing something quite ordinary – shaving. This is an ordinary thing done by ordinary people. But their conversation shows just how extraordinary this ordinary thing is for both blind and sighted persons. It is through the ordinary stuff of everyday life that the extraordinary and mysterious character of the human condition is revealed.

2

What Is Blindness?

The most dramatic expression of blindness is its occurrence in a human being. Perhaps the most dramatic fictional portrayal of blindness occurs in H.G. Wells's short story 'The Country of the Blind' (1927, 123–46). Both of these expressions represent a story of blindness. The former is a story in that blindness is experienced and revealed in the life of an individual, while Wells's fictional account tells a story of how blindness is conceived of in society. Fictional or not, blindness is always revealed through narration and is always dramatic.

Blindness is always experienced in the midst of sightedness. People are either born blind into a world organized by sight or lose their sight in the same world. Most people are not blind, and the meaning of blindness is understood within the social context of its rare occurrence. Thus the meaning of blindness is wrapped in the cloak of its immersion in a 'sighted world.' This immersion is always dramatic.

Wells's story is particularly revealing in that he reverses this dramatic immersion. He tells of the adventure of Nunez, a sighted person, who literally stumbles into a valley inhabited solely by blind persons. This country of the blind had come into being generations ago. No one had ever seen it. Everyone had heard about it. Nunez was the first sighted person to stumble upon it.

The story goes that many years ago some people found themselves trapped in a valley isolated in the mountains of Ecuador. These people were cut off from all other civilization. A disease caused these inhabitants to go blind. This disease was genetic and, over many generations of isolation, caused blindness in all of the inhabitants. Moreover, this passage of time meant that this entire population lived as though blindness was normal. They knew nothing of sight and nothing of blindness since the two could only be known if they existed together.

Earlier generations did remember their seeing days. But over time, the wise ones of the country of the blind dismissed these stories as fantasy and myth. They replaced these imaginings with those that come from the ears and finger tips. Soon this country was organized solely by senses other than sight. Religion and philosophy, government and administration, as well as work and recreation were all organized with touch, hearing, and smell as the primary modes of knowing and believing. It was upon this country that Nunez stumbled.

Nunez was guiding a party through the mountains when he accidentally fell. Thousands of feet and many hours later, he found himself on the outskirts of the country of the blind. He was hurt, tired, and hungry, and glad to see people. In his exuberance, he waved at them in an attempt to get their attention, but none was forthcoming. He then noticed that the houses of these people were oddly formed, without windows, and were spattered with oddly matching coloured plaster. 'The good man who did that,' he thought, 'must have been as blind as a bat' (1927, 128). As is the case for many people, this was merely a manner of speaking for Nunez. He did not believe it; but the reality soon struck him. He tried yet again to get their attention, but could not. 'The fools must be blind' (ibid., 129).

Finally, Nunez called out and then approached the people in the country of the blind. Nunez tried to tell them that he could see. But words such as *see, sight,* and *look* had no meaning to the people. Try as he might, Nunez could not get his sight across to them. The people in the country of the blind, thought Nunez, were extremely odd. For their part, they thought he was newly born of the rocks and thus ill-formed. Nunez had much to learn about the country and a long way to go before he became a well-formed citizen.

But this was not Nunez's opinion. He thought himself far superior to the people of the country of the blind since, after all, he could see. Nunez reminded himself of the adage 'In the Country of the Blind the One-eyed Man is King' (ibid., 129). He tried to convince these citizens of his superior ability and of the existence of a 'sighted world' beyond their country. They would have nothing of this. To the citizens, Nunez was a blasphemer.

Nunez was not accustomed to organizing his world without sight. As he tried to convince the citizens of the country of the blind of his superior ability, he continually stumbled over things, including the citizens:

... Pedro [a citizen] went first and took Nunez by the hand to lead him to the houses.

He drew his hand away. 'I can see,' he said.

'See?' said Correa [another citizen].

'Yes, see,' said Nunez, turning towards him, and stumbling against Pedro's pail.

'His senses are still imperfect,' said the third blind man. 'He stumbles, and talks unmeaning words. Lead him by the hand.'

'As you will,' said Nunez, and was led, along, laughing. (ibid., 131)

But Nunez's laughter soon turned to tears. He came to realize that his sight disabled him in this country. Nunez was incompetent and could not get along without blindness. Nunez had to adapt to the 'blind world' in much the same way that blind persons must adapt to the 'sighted world.' Like many blind persons, Nunez cried.

The medical expert in the country of the blind developed both a diagnosis and a solution to Nunez's problem. The diagnosis was the following:

Those queer things that are called eyes, and which exist to make an agreeable soft depression in the face, are diseased ... in such a way as to affect his brain. They are greatly distended, he has eyelashes, and his eyelids move, and consequently his brain is in a state of constant irritation and distraction. (ibid., 142)

The solution was 'to remove these irritant bodies' (ibid., 143). Finally, the cure. But Nunez was not happy. Despite his incompetence, he did not want to be blind. He longed for his sighted world.

During this time, Nunez fell in love with one of the citizens, Medina-sarote. She loved him and wanted nothing more than to live with Nunez in the country of the blind. For this, however, Nunez would have to be cured. As disagreeable as this was to Nunez, love made him submit to the cure.

Wells wrote two different endings to this story. Different as they are, they amount to the same thing. The first depicts Nunez as escaping from the country of the blind despite his love. However, he is not able to complete his escape and thus dies. Nunez preferred death to blindness.

The second ending brings death to the country of the blind. On the eve of his cure, Nunez notices a crack in the mountain. Realizing that the mountain will fall and bury the country, Nunez becomes panic-stricken. He tries to convince the citizens of what he saw. They do not believe him. There is a resounding crack as the mountain continues to split. The citizens interpret this as a warning from their gods, who are warning them of the evil of sight, which Nunez is now expressing in a wild and desperate way. He wants to save the country from disaster, but the citizens think Nunez is the disaster. As the mountain falls, Nunez escapes with his love, Medina-sarote, clinging to him. They survive and continue their life in Nunez's home.

Both endings are equally dramatic. Blindness brings ultimate disaster. Choosing blindness over sightedness results in death.

Wells's story depicts the meeting of blindness and sightedness. He reverses the typical form of the meeting by immersing sightedness in blindness. This results in death. Blindness acts as a reminder of what is lost. What is lost is ability, the love of looking, the knowledge that seeing brings; in short, a version of life itself. This loss is dramatically depicted by Wells as he immerses sightedness in blindness. 'In the Country of the Blind the One-eyed Man is Lost.'

But what of the typical meeting of blindness and sightedness? What story is told when blindness is immersed in sightedness? How do we respond to Wells's story? One response is to tell another story. Every story of blindness is a depiction of what blindness is. Wells gives us one such depiction. I want now to tell a story of a blind person in the country of the sighted.

THE BLINK

He coughed. 'Dry throat, water,' he said in a raspy voice. He lifted the glass to his lips and drank what was left of the water. 'There, that's better,' he said. 'We're almost done. This is the last page. It looks like the conclusion.'

He didn't usually like what he read to her, but this was different. He really liked this story. The *Country of the Blind*, he thought, what an interesting idea. This H.G. Wells guy must have had quite an imagination. Imagine, Nunez, a sighted guy, stumbling into this country. No one could see! And, yet, they lived and found ways to do everything! Fascinating, he thought. Then, how romantic, he fell in love with Medina-sarote and took her out of the country just as the mountain fell on it. Exciting or what?

He glanced at the last page again. And his eyes were drawn to the last thing on the page. 'It may be beautiful,' said Medina-sarote, 'but it must be very terrible to *see*.' For some reason, he looked across the table at Jenny. Man, he thought.

'That's better,' he repeated. 'Well, let's finish it.'

'Well,' he said, 'that's it, that's the end.' He placed the pages on the low table in front of him and looked at her, trying to discern her response. He did, after all, want her thoughts on the story he had just read.

She sat quietly, almost pensively, gazing slightly upward and biting gently on her bottom lip. Many people had asked her about this story in the past, but this was the first time she had heard it. She recalled that her high-school teacher had told her about this story years ago and she remembered, too, how her teacher said that being blind was only different because most people were sighted. Even back then, when she was fifteen years old, she often wondered what things would be like if most people were blind.

He interrupted her thoughts. 'What do you think?'

'Oh,' she said, fixing her gaze on him, 'it was good, it was good.'

The memory of her high-school teacher drifted back to her once more. This teacher was the first one ever to even raise the possibility that being blind wasn't so different, at least the first one Jenny believed. Almost on its own, at least that's what it appeared like to him, her gaze moved to some distant place. She began touching her white cane, which was folded on her lap. The warmth of the rubber handle was quite a contrast to the coolness of the three aluminum segments of the cane's shaft. She almost grinned as she now recalled the security she felt when she clutched that rubber handle for the first time years ago when she was only eight. The same sense of security flooded over her now.

Cane directly in front of your right foot. She concentrated as hard as she could. *Index finger of your right hand pointing straight down the cane. The cane is actually an extension of your index finger. Step forward with your left foot and, at the same time, and with your index finger, move the cane in an arc directly in front of your left foot.* Her other fingers moved slightly around the warm rubber handle of her cane. *Then forward with your right foot. At the same time arc your cane in front of your right foot. Now concentrate on the movement. This technique means that your long cane, your long index finger, will have simultaneously moved in front of every step and it will let you know if anything is in the way.*

Concentrate! Concentrate! I have the rubber handle. This helps.

Her mind suddenly returned and she fixed her gaze on him once more.

'It's an interesting story,' he said.

'It is, it really is,' she replied.

'You know,' he said, 'I sometimes wonder what it's like for you. I mean, I sometimes wonder what you see. You know, is it all black? Is it all white?'

Having heard this question all of her life and, to her, what seemed like a million times, she laughed. 'I don't know. Black or white, I don't know.'

Feeling just a little silly, he said, 'Yeah, I'm sorry, I guess not.'

'Don't be sorry,' she quickly said. 'You know what it's like? Here, make a fist.' She held her fist up for him to see.

'Okay.'

'Now put it behind your back,' she said.

'Yeah.'

'Now,' she said, drawing out the word, 'pretend your fist is your eyes.'

'What?' he asked.

'You know, pretend your fist is your eyes.'

'Okay,' he said.

'Now,' again drawing the word out, she asked, 'what do you see?'

He reached over the little table and touched her with his fistful of eyes. He laughed and said, 'I get it, I get it.'

She gently touched his hand with hers and joined him in his laughter. Suddenly, the memory was back.

Concentrate! Concentrate! Well, it's as hard as a rock. Jeez, hang on to that handle. It's amazing how hard this is. I can feel it, I can feel it! Oops, what? That's not hard.

Remember to concentrate. You're veering slightly to your left and your cane is picking up some grass at the edge of the sidewalk.

I get it, I get it.

Don't panic. It's fine. You just have to correct yourself. Square to the edge of the sidewalk. There, you're fine.

I'm okay. My finger, I need this handle! Okay, I'm touching the sidewalk again. Funny how different that grass felt. I need the handle. Are we around the block yet?

No, no. Remember what I said, we need to make four left-hand turns. Remember the curbs.

Oh yeah, I forgot. Just keep going and then I'll touch the curb. This handle is good.

You're doing fine.

Around the block, around the block. He says I'm supposed to end up right back at my house. I sort of know what he means. I wonder how big those curbs are. Gotta remember my house when I get back here. Okay, okay, I gotta think. Touching, touching. The handle, I love this handle.

Interrupting her thoughts once more, he said, 'That's terrific. It must be that way, it's like nothing! I never said this before, but I really do think about it a lot.'

'About blindness?' she asked almost surprised.

'Yeah,' he continued. 'But actually it's more about you, you know, I think more about what it must be like for *you* to be blind.'

'I didn't know that,' she said, fixing her gaze on his even more intently than before. 'You've never mentioned that before. After all these years, you never said you thought about it.'

'I know,' he replied, dropping his voice ever so slightly. 'I mean, I know you very well. That's not the problem. I just sometimes feel ... well, I don't want to treat you like a curiosity.'

'Are you curious?' she asked.

'I am,' he replied. 'But I'm a little embarrassed about it.'

'Don't be,' she said smiling. 'Think about it, I'm always asking you about what you see.'

He paused for a moment and said, 'I know, but somehow that's different. You only ask me because you want to know what things are like.'

This time not smiling at him, she said, 'Yeah, I know.'

Once more her memory penetrated her thought. It took her back once again to when she got her first white cane and when she received, what they referred to as, 'orientation and mobility lessons.' The school never provided these lessons. *That school!* The thought of it made her shudder. She really didn't like it and was very happy to be back home again.

There was absolutely no reason for her to go to that school, at least that's what she thought. Fifteen hundred miles away from home. At the time, she had no idea what that meant. But having to get to the school on an aeroplane and coming home only during school holidays and summer vacation soon made her realize that, no matter how many miles away from home the school was, it was far away. Two years of this, she hated it!

She shoved the memory from her mind with such a force that it jerked her attention back to him.

'Are you okay?' he asked.

She shook her head and said, 'Oh yeah, I'm sorry, I was just thinking about that stupid school.'

'University?' he asked quizzically.

'No, no,' she said quickly, 'that blind school. Anyway, so you think about my blindness?' He said he did and went on talking about how not seeing anything from birth was like seeing nothing. It seemed, to her, that he was quite taken with this idea. He kept speaking about it as though he needed to understand it but, somehow, could not wrap his thoughts around it.

Finally, she said, 'It's not that much different for me. I have just as much trouble trying to understand what it must be like to see.'

'I suppose you're right,' he said in that slow way of speaking that often understands itself as insightful wisdom.

She wasn't sure whether or not it was his voice that triggered it, but her memory, now acting completely independently of her, drew her back in time. Her memory pushed the voice of that social worker into her mind. She remembered that first visit as if it was actually happening now.

'Jenny, Jen.' Her mother was calling. 'Jenny your worker's here.'

'Worker,' she thought, 'worker, that's funny.'

Her mother's voice again, this time more loudly. 'Come on Jen, Judy's here, your worker's here.'

'Is she working now?' Jenny thought. 'She couldn't be,' Jenny concluded, 'because Judy would work, well, at work, and she was here. So she wasn't working.'

My worker, your worker, his worker, her worker. She didn't know it at the time but these phrases would penetrate her consciousness, indeed become part of her very being. Saying 'my worker' or 'your worker' would, for Jenny, become as natural as saying 'my jacket' or 'my shoes' or even as natural as saying 'my hair.' The 'worker,' yes, the worker, she thought. Yes, we need workers. That's what I'm like, I'm like a person who needs a worker. I need to be worked on. They work on me. They work with me. They do work to me. Yes, she thought, they are workers. I'm like their project. Where do they go when they go to work? They go here, they go there. They go wherever people like me are. I'm here, they work. Work, work, work. They may work, but I am work.

It suddenly struck her that there would be lots of work for workers to do in the country of the blind, if there was such a place. Yes, she laughed to herself, Judy would be very busy in such a country. Work, work, work. There would be lots to do. Judy would be even busier than Nunez, she thought.

Somewhere off in the distance she heard him ask, 'What are you thinking about?'

'Oh, nothing really,' she wistfully replied. 'It's just interesting how many sighties are curious about blind people.'

'Listen,' he said, 'I'm sorry, I'm really sorry.'

'There you go again,' she laughed, 'being sorry. You know, I feel much better when you are curious about me than when you feel sorry for me.'

He laughed, and touched her again.

Her memory yanked her back once more, and Jenny remembered the touch of Judy's hand on her shoulder.

'This is Judy your worker, remember?' her mother asked. Jenny didn't, but she said she did. Judy was happy to see her but then, in some strange way, it seemed as if Judy was talking to her mother even though it sounded like she was talking to her. Jenny was surprised by this. 'Was Judy working now?' she thought. Maybe my mother's working too. Maybe they're both working.

Judy seemed very very bubbly. There was much, much work to be done. You're just at the beginning of integration and Jenny is ... you are ... one of the first. As a parent, her mother must be very excited and proud. 'As a parent ...,' Jenny thought, as what else could she be excited and proud?

Jenny wasn't sure about this 'much, much work.' She knew most of the kids in her neighbourhood, they were her friends. 'At last,' she thought, she would be going to school with them. Is that what Judy meant by work? There was the school work. But Jenny knew she would be doing that and didn't think there would be any left over for Judy to do. Maybe Judy would do her homework. Is that it? Would Judy always be here, at her home, waiting for her to come home with her homework? 'God, I hope not,' she thought.

'I think you're right,' he said after a long pause. 'I mean, it's good for people to be curious about one another, especially friends. You're right, I'm curious about your blindness and, you know, it's no big deal. After all, you're a person, just like me and because you happen to be blind' – he stressed this last part – 'I'm curious, it's no big deal.'

You just happen to be blind. Her memory took over her thoughts once again. Jenny remembered the first time she heard this. It was actually Judy, her worker, who had said this to her for the first time. *You just happen to be blind.* It wasn't much consolation at the time.

'Remember that you're a person,' Judy had told her, 'blindness is only a small part of you.' Jenny certainly didn't feel that way. It seemed that blindness was the biggest part of her.

This time Jenny took control and snapped herself back to where she was. 'Do you think, do you think that Medina ...' She then stammered slightly, trying to remember the last part of Medina's name. She found this amusing since she was often complimented on her great memory. 'Do you think that Medina was curious about the people in Nunez's home country?'

'That never occurred to me,' he said.

She didn't understand why, but Jenny's memory took her back to a beach in Vancouver. She remembered sitting on one of those big logs that the tide often drifts up to the shore.

A little boy, or a little girl, Jenny did not know which, suddenly spoke to her and asked her what was wrong. She said that nothing was wrong. The child said that she looked funny. Jenny laughed and told the child that she was blind. She must have had her eyes closed because the child said that she should open her eyes. That wouldn't matter, she still couldn't see, Jenny told the child. 'Well, go to a doctor,' the child advised. Jenny said that that wouldn't help either. Seeming satisfied, the child said, 'Okay' and left.

'She must have been curious,' he said, interrupting her thoughts again. 'Nunez's country was the complete opposite to what she had known for all of her life so far.'

'She must have been,' Jenny agreed, 'but there's not even a hint of it in the story. I don't find this surprising somehow.'

'What do you mean?' he asked.

'Well,' she said, 'I said I was curious about your sight, but, quite honestly, I'm not sure that I was until now. I think it was that story that actually made me curious.'

He leaned slightly forward and reached out his hand to touch her. Changing his mind, for what reason he wasn't sure, and, in the intonation of that type of question that really isn't, he said, 'You mean you never were curious about sight? You never thought about what people see?'

'I suppose in one way, but not really,' she said. 'I honestly don't remember when I first became aware of the fact that people see. They just do, people see. It seems like that awareness has always been with me.' To say that he looked at her would be to minimize this look. What he actually looked at were her hands, her arms and shoulders, her white cane, in fact, he seemed to look at her by looking everywhere except into her eyes. In that sense of surprise that comes with self-realization, he caught himself doing so. He wasn't sure why he was surprised, but he was. At that imperceptibly brief moment between self-realization and surprise, he very purposely caused his eyes to look into hers. At the moment his eyes met hers, he wondered whether or not she could see him. 'That's curious,' he simultaneously thought and said aloud.

'That's true,' she said. 'It seems like I've always had the impression that you can see everything, you know, that sighted people can see everything. The funny thing about this, now that I think about it, is that I don't even know what everything is except, whatever it is, you can see it. I guess that's why I've never been curious. You can see everything, it's no big deal, it's no mystery.'

'But that story seemed to make you curious,' he said.

In control once more, her memory returned. This time, and surprising her not a little, Jenny's memory returned her to her first actual encounter with death. She had read about it before, saw movies about it, and, like everyone else, had even thought about it. But this was the first time she had actually encountered it.

She remembered her age, she was seventeen. Jenny recalled how she had headed out to meet a friend, Tom, at a cafe. She remembered feeling the slight flow of cool air coming from her left, and she knew she had just passed the buildings and was approaching the curb at the cross-street. Jenny's memory seemed to play with her again.

Concentrate! Concentrate! But just then, a voice, a voice of a friend. She stopped immediately while, at the same time, storing the fact in her memory that she was quite near the curb. Jenny greeted her friend enthusiastically. After her friend told Jenny that Sarah, another friend, was also there, Jenny granted the same enthusiastic greeting to Sarah. Just then, and even now Jenny shuddered, her friend explained that Sarah's baby sister had just died.

At that moment, Jenny felt the explosion that comes with the rush of the penetration of the multitude of feelings into the self. She told Sarah that she was sorry. She felt a genuine urge to hug Sarah but, at that moment, the disorientation of the kaleidoscope of feelings passed from her soul into her body. Jenny reached her arms out, almost wildly, dropping her cane in the process. She had no idea where Sarah was, where the curb was, and, for an indescribable instant of terror, where she was. Sarah grasped Jenny and both sobbed softly into one another.

It wasn't until later, much later, perhaps even two or three months later, that Jenny realized that this encounter left her with some anger. Jenny had read the books and had even seen the movies, the ones she liked to call 'TV cause movies,' that describe the anger that comes when someone close dies. But Jenny was not close to Sarah's baby sister. Of course, she felt tremendous sorrow for Sarah and felt the contradiction when someone so young dies. But this wasn't why she was angry.

Jenny knew why she was angry and knew, too, that there was nothing she could do about it. This is probably why she had put off thinking about it for quite some time. The anger came to her now though, cloaked as it was, in the memory of her first encounter with death.

Jenny met his gaze, and, for her, this wasn't just an expression since she consciously tried to do so. 'You know, I don't think I was curious about sight until now, but there were times when I thought you sighties were really lucky and I even felt a little jealous and even angry.'

'You mean because we can see?' he asked.

'Yeah, because you can see so much, you can see everything!' she said. 'Geez, you can even see how people feel.'

Somewhat bewildered, he asked, 'What do you mean?'

'Well,' she said, 'there's facial expressions, the eyes, windows to the soul, and all that shit. I mean that's a real advantage, seeing that stuff.'

This time he intentionally and, even intensely, looked into her eyes, although for what he wasn't sure. For a moment, he got the eerie impression that her eyes were more like mirrors than windows. He wondered whose soul he was looking into. 'I guess that is a real advantage,' he said, 'but you know ...'

'Of course it is,' she interrupted. 'You know when someone's feeling shitty just by looking at them and then you don't make a fool of yourself by talking as if the whole world is happy.' She paused for a moment and looked down. As suddenly as she had interrupted him, Jenny snapped her eyes back into his. 'Now that I think about it, I am curious about sight and maybe I always was. What the fuck do you see when you look at someone's face?'

He was so startled by her question, filled with fury as it was, that this time he did touch her but more to soothe her than anything else. 'Whoa,' he said, 'what are you so pissed off about?'

'Well it's quite an advantage,' she replied with just as much fire in her voice as before, 'it's quite an advantage to see somebody's mood. I'd sure like to do that once in a while.'

'Yeah, but don't forget,' he said, 'you've got amazing hearing and you can tell what they're feeling just by the sound of their voice.'

'Oh please,' she said disgustedly.

'It's true, it's true!' he exclaimed laughing.

The fire in her voice now reduced to a smoulder, she said, 'That's sort of true. But, you know, you have to hear the voice first. *You* can just look at someone's face and, even from a long distance, you can tell.'

'Well, I'm not going to sit here and tell you that seeing isn't an advantage, that's for sure,' he said with a somewhat definite tone.

'No, I know,' she said, reassuring him. Jenny then laughed. 'You know those people, you know the ones, the ones who say, "Oh I know you're blind but I can't see anything without my glasses."'

He joined Jenny in her laughter.

'And then there's the ones,' she continued, 'you know, "Well, we all have a disability."'

He didn't find this as humorous but, still, he continued to laugh.

'Sometimes, when people say that to me, I feel like saying, "Yeah, well you should try blindness on for size."'

Laughing all the while, he said, 'Then they'd really know what it's like.'

'Yeah,' she said in a somewhat cynical but thoughtful sort of way. Then her memory took up its game once more. Jenny fiddled with her folded white cane as she remembered.

Concentrate! Concentrate! The rubber handle feels good. I like it. I can make it, I can make it. Just three more blocks. Damn! Is it two? No, I've already gone four. Or, did I go three? Damn, I don't know! I don't know! Concentrate! Concentrate! Try to remember. Try! You've got to remember! Right, right, okay, just relax. Everything's okay. Remember, that last block has that funny stuff. What do they call it? Oh shit, I forget. Oh yeah, cobblestones. Great, cobblestones, then turn right.

That's better, just relax. This feels good. My finger, my warm handle. Touch the sidewalk, touch the ground, keep touching. Touch the world.

Why the hell did I wear heels? It's night-time, dummy. Time to go to the pub. Everyone's there, you're late enough. Be cool, be cool. You can always take a cab home. It'll be late, they won't think anything of it. Lots of people take cabs when it's late. It's no big deal. Geez, don't worry about it now. Concentrate! Concentrate!

'Do you think,' he asked, interrupting her thoughts again and, yet again, doing so unknowingly, 'do you think that being sighted is terrible like Medina-sarote said?'

She was surprised that he had remembered Medina's full name, so much so that she had forgotten his question. 'Pardon?' she asked.

He met her gaze and repeated his question. This time, however, he looked into her eyes intending to see her. He could not help wondering what she saw and, equally as strange to him, he could not help seeing himself in her eyes. What he saw was that he was uncomfortable asking her this question. When he took a second look, he saw that he was actually more embarrassed than uncomfortable. What he couldn't see, however, was why he was embarrassed. After all, this idea that being sighted was terrible was not his. It was in the story and that's where Jenny had heard it first. He didn't raise this idea. But still, he was asking her about it. Still looking into her eyes, he blinked.

'That's what got me thinking,' she said, not really answering his question. 'Medina, Medina, ah, ah, what's her name?'

'Sarote,' he replied.

'Right,' she continued. 'That's the thing, that's the thing I wonder about. She never asked about his sight before. Nowhere did she tell Nunez that she was curious about seeing. Oh yeah, she liked him talking about flowers and stuff like that, but ... and, did you notice that from the time she arrived at Nunez's country till the end of the story, absolutely nothing about sight!'

'That's true,' he said, now looking everywhere except into her eyes.

'Not once,' she went on, 'not once did Medina, ah, ... she never said anything about Nunez's country. But Nunez, well, most of the story talked about what he thought of her country. Lots about blindness but almost nothing about sight. Well, nothing directly anyway. But I guess that's what it's like.'

Noticing that he was looking into her eyes once again, he blinked and asked, 'That's what *what's* like?'

This time intending to answer him, she said, 'There's lots said about blindness. Many people are curious. And, the ones who say the most and the ones who are most curious are sighted! You never hear too much said about sight. But even when you do, sighted people say it. I mean, sighties have been telling me about sight all of my life. Come to think of it, they've been telling me about blindness all of my life too!'

'They tell you about sight?' he said surprised.

'You know,' she said, 'I've always been told it's a "sighted world." That's what it's like, that's reality. You have to fit in Jenny. You have to adapt to it. You have to learn your orientation and mobility. Here's how you cook on a stove. It's not so bad Jenny, they say, any university book you need will be on tape or in Braille. Remember to make eye contact and smile. That's what sighted people do. It goes on and on and on.'

'Yeah, I see what you mean,' he said, blinking more than ever now.

'I used to believe them, you know,' she said, 'but now I'm not so sure.' Then once again, her memory.

Jenny remembered gasping her feelings to her mother through her sobs. She was screaming at her mother but not because she was angry at her. Oh, she was angry all right but not really with her mother. Jenny knew her mother had something to do with it, but she was angry more at the rest of them.

'They all hate me,' she screamed. 'They all stare at me. It's like a zoo!' Jenny's mother tried to assure her that the students at her new school were not staring at her, but with no success. No one joked with her, no one teased her, in fact, they were, and always were, nice to her. It's not that they weren't nice to each other but they joked and teased with each other. They laughed and had fun. But not with her, oh no, not with her. Jenny hated this school more than the blind school. At least at the blind school, everyone was like her. We all joked, we all teased, we had fun.

A sudden shudder brought her back to him. It was her turn to blink and she said, 'Sometimes I think he assigned that story to us on purpose.'

'You think your professor put Wells's story on the reading list because you're blind?' he asked.

She felt herself blinking and paused slightly. 'Not exactly,' she said. 'Don't forget, it's this dumb social psych. course. Lots of experts, everyone's an expert on something. Then, then if you're the thing, well, then you're certainly the expert. You know what I mean?'

'I think so,' he said.

'I mean, there must be over a hundred of us in this class,' she continued. 'He just lectures. He never just picks one person out, like, he never just asks one person a question. But this time, this time, he asks me! He comes right out and asks! He just says, "What's it like Jenny?"'

'Really!' he exclaimed.

It seemed as though she was in the midst of forming a word when her memory erased it from her lips and once more took her back to her childhood.

Concentrate! Concentrate! Around the block. Now I don't know! Around the block. Think! Think! The rubber handle, that's nice. Just relax. Around the block, I don't know. Around the block. Concentrate! You're supposed to get back home again.

What's this? What's this? Yikes! What's this? That's not grass. Touch it, touch it. My finger, touch it. What is this? Use your whole hand. Wood? What is this? Well, it's a telephone pole on the side of the sidewalk. A telephone pole! Wood, I think. Round too. Reaching, reaching, reaching. It's tall. I can't reach anymore. It's really high. Does it go as high as the sky? No, it might be about thirty feet high. Thirty feet high! What's that? Touch it. Touch it. I see, you mean the sky starts at thirty feet? Ground, sky. Touch it, touch it. Around the block. Concentrate!

'Yeah,' she said, coming back to him, 'stories about blindness, I'm blind, I'm the expert. Can you believe it?'

He looked in her eyes and saw that he was intrigued. 'What did you say to him?'

This time Jenny leaned slightly forward, grasped the rubber handle of her white cane, and said, 'Believe it or not, honest to God, I told him I didn't know.'

His intrigue seemed to bring him closer. Just then he realized that he must be displaying the same sort of intrigue that Jenny's professor had. For an instant, he wondered if Jenny saw his intrigue. He knew she didn't, but he leaned back anyway and, purposely clearing his throat, he asked, 'What did he say?'

'Nothing just then,' she replied. 'You know me, I went on. I told him that I thought blindness was a country.'

Her other life, or so it seemed to her, beckoned her once again, and she turned, gently this time, to face it.

The book felt good. Jenny opened the plain brown cover which was thinner than the pages and silently began to read.

Without a jerk this time, and with no interruption, she came back to him as gently as she had left.

'Do you really think blindness is a country?' he asked.

'Yes,' she said with a glimmer of sadness that could be seen only in her voice, 'yes, I think so.'

Their eyes met and, in that meeting, rested. He looked at her, and, for the first time, he saw that she was looking at him.

Both 'The Country of the Blind' and 'The Blink' raise the question of blindness. Answers to this question are revealed in the telling of these stories. They provide a portrayal of blindness through a narrative account of its meaning. Both stories begin with some answer to the question of the meaning of blindness and weave this meaning through the telling of the story.

Sightedness is a key antagonist in both stories. Both depict the meaning of blindness as something which results from the interaction of seeing and not seeing. Blindness is born of the meeting of these two antagonists. Each time these antagonists meet, the question of blindness is simultaneously asked and answered.

'Country' is an interesting metaphor. It suggests a geography and a place. Countries are made up of a 'people' – a people with customs, habits, and a language. People of one country are distinct from those of another by virtue of these things as well as by social and political organization. Stories of blindness tell of the meeting of two countries. These stories always raise the question of blindness and its place in the country of sightedness.

Thus the question What is blindness? is raised each and every time we meet a blind person, talk about blindness, or even think about it. This question is most often raised tacitly, but it is, nevertheless, raised. Karatheodoris (1982, 31) addresses this issue. He says:

What is blindness? This question has received many different answers. Some say that blindness is a tragedy; others, that it is a medical or technical problem. Still others claim that blindness is a social problem. No matter how we conceive of blindness, however, one thing is certain. Our conception will influence the way in which we orient to blind and visually impaired persons. Thus, no matter how we answer the question, What is blindness?, our answer will influence our conduct and our social relations. The way in which a blind person himself answers this question will influence how he conceives of himself as well as how others conceive of him.

If Karatheodoris is right, and I believe that he is, we should be able to examine various conceptions of blindness with an eye to understanding the sorts of everyday relations that these conceptions produce. The reverse is also true; an examination of everyday relations to blindness can tell us something about the conceptions that animate these relations.

Karatheodoris *himself* implicitly gives us a conception of blindness. Blindness is a tragedy, a medical or technical problem, a social problem. Blindness *is a* problem. But surely this conception of blindness does not belong only to Karatheodoris. The problem of blindness that he raises reflects his own culture's conception that, in one way or another, blindness is a problem. It is to this conception of blindness that our deliberations now turn.

Saying that blindness is a problem seems somewhat superfluous. The very word already suggests a problem, and, in fact, we use it as one way to show that a problem exists. We say, for example, that someone is 'blind to the facts' or that someone 'turns a blind eye,' or we say, 'What's the matter ump, are you blind?' Such everyday expressions are used metaphorically to suggest the idea of 'something missing' or the idea of 'lack,' 'inability,' or 'incompetence.' Being 'blind to the facts' suggests that something is missing, namely facts. 'Turning a blind eye' suggests a lack of attention. And calling a baseball umpire 'blind' is one way to suggest inability and incompetence.

But these expressions suggest even more than lack or inability. They imply that things *should* be otherwise: we should look at the facts; we should pay attention; and baseball umpires should possess ability – they should not act *as if* they are blind. Everyday usage of the word *blind* shows how a problem is built into the word itself, and this usage also shows how this problem is assumed in the very speaking and hearing of the word.

Blindness conceived of as lack presupposes the problem that comes with a disruption to the usual-state-of-affairs. What blindness disrupts is the usual-state-of-affairs we know as sight. It is this disruptive character of blindness that allows for the conception of blindness as lack and that points to the understanding that things *should* be otherwise.

We say of some people that they have 'gone blind,' or of others that they were 'born blind,' or of others that they are 'losing' or have 'lost' their sight. Again, we can see how these expressions suggest that things should have been otherwise. 'Going blind,' 'losing sight,' and the like, tell us a story of what life ought to or should be like. These expressions tell us what life should be by implicitly telling us that people should not go blind, they should not lose their sight, or they should not be born without it. Words such as 'gone,' 'lost,' and 'losing,' when used in relation to sight, point to the value of that which is gone or lost; they make implicit reference to the value of the state-of-affairs we call sight.

That sight is considered valuable is shown in how we speak about its absence. The conception of blindness as a problem turns on the value of sight, and, as a problem, blindness finds its very possibility in the way that sight and blindness interact to produce the meaning of both. The interaction of sight and blindness is the interaction between that which is valuable and that which is not. We value sight and when we lose something valuable, or if we never had it in the first place, we have a problem.

It would be nonsensical to speak of losing something which is not valuable. Imagine saying that we have lost our trash or that we have lost our toothpick. Losing trash or toothpicks is, indeed, not conceived of as a problem or, for that matter, as a loss. Imagine, on the other hand, losing a large quantity of money or a diamond ring. Undoubtedly, these are losses. They are losses, however, that do not in any way compare to the loss of sight. We speak of loss only when the object to which it refers is deemed valuable. As a corollary, we speak of gain only when we acquire or reacquire something we consider valuable.

We can now see why so much importance is placed on programs such as sight restoration and conservation. We can understand the value of blindness prevention programs. These programs are generated under the auspices of doing what can be done to prevent the loss of something valuable – sight. Whenever we deem something valuable, we take some form of action oriented to preventing its loss. This action is oriented to the possibility of the loss of that which is valuable. The possibility of blindness reminds us that sight is valuable and that action should be taken to retain it and to prevent its loss.

The loss of a valued object is often described in terms that depict both the value of the object lost and the worthless nature of what results from this loss. When someone loses their mind, they are mentally ill. When someone loses their fortune, they are penniless. When someone loses their sight, they are blind. A sound mind, a fortune, and sight are not spoken of in terms of loss since they are themselves valued. We do not say of persons who have had their sight restored that they have *lost their blindness.* Instead, we say that their sight was restored or that they regained their sight. Programs do not exist, except in the country of the blind, for the prevention of sightedness. In the country of the sighted, blindness is not valued, and action is not oriented to its potential loss or acquisition. In this country, blindness is conceived of as a problem. Blindness represents the sheer necessity of living a life without the particular value of seeing.

The problem of blindness is often understood in terms of 'trouble.' When a problem is conceived of as trouble, the value bestowed upon the troublesome thing is twofold: first, the troublesome thing is given the negative value that is attributed to *any* troublesome thing; and second, there is value, albeit implicit and indirect, insofar as any troublesome thing puts us in mind of the value it presupposes. Blindness often puts us in mind of the value of sight, and trouble has value insofar as it reminds us of the very thing that it troubles. It is no wonder that the ways in which blindness is spoken about in everyday life fail to address the value of blindness. This is why, from this perspective, blindness has no value except to remind us, those of us who can see, of our good fortune. Hence, the expression 'There but for the grace of God go I.' It is not surprising that this perspective can only generate medical, rehabilitative, and educational remedies for blindness, as well as prevention-of-blindness programs.

Clearly, blindness represents adversity. We can see that adversity is conceived of as trouble that should ideally be prevented but, failing prevention, should be remedied. From this perspective, adversity means nothing more and nothing less than a problem conceived as trouble. This is not to say that blindness is not an adverse condition since, for many, blindness is a traumatic experience. Its onset often disrupts, in an overwhelming way, not only the routines of everyday life but also a sense of worth, well-being, and self-esteem. The onset of blindness means that the taken-for-granted ways of looking and seeing, as well as the ways of conducting a life, can no longer be relied upon since they no longer exist. Blindness also means a disruption to the tacit ways we typically think of ourselves and our rela- tion to others; it disrupts how we conceive of the reality of a world we have come to know and trust. Blindness represents adversity as it is often experienced as a disruption of reality, a reality that is taken for granted and experienced from a standpoint that is sound, firm, and unchanging. Blindness is often experienced as an adverse imposition onto a life that has always been relied upon even though this reliance has been assumed and presupposed to be 'just there' for us to count on and unthoughtfully know.

The problem with adversity conceived as trouble is that it does not change things. Blindness does not change the understanding that sight is the normal-state-of-affairs, nor does it change the understanding that sight is the best and most valuable way of looking and seeing. It is easy to see that, from this standpoint, blindness is a trouble that, like any other trouble, must be eradicated or, failing that, coped with. Whether coping methods involve rehabilitation, adjustment-to-blindness programs, or the like, these methods represent ways and means for sustaining the value of sight. It is often said that a blind person must learn to cope within a 'sighted world.' Even though those who say this intend the expression 'sighted world' as a description of the world, this expression is one method available to them for achieving a world they can take for granted and implicitly know.

The expression 'sighted world' is a metaphor that contributes to achieving the interpretation of adversity as trouble. This expression is spoken and heard only in the midst of blindness. Blindness does not change things. It has no influence. The expression 'sighted world' reminds blind persons that they are living in the country of the sighted and that they must learn its language, customs, and folk-ways. There is no 'multiculturalism' in this country when it comes to blindness. Regardless of who goes blind or, for that matter, how many, the expression 'sighted world' reminds us of the unchanging, eternal, and thus valuable nature of what it means to see. This was the memory that Nunez brought with him when he stumbled into the country of the blind.

Unlike blindness, sightedness is understood as trouble-free. The 'sighted world' now becomes a realm where life can be carried on in a taken-for-granted way insofar as the naturalness and, therefore, value of this realm are not questioned. But blindness introduces trouble into this realm in that it makes it necessary for sightedness to look upon itself and discover ways that it can accommodate blindness without destroying the natural and taken-for-granted character of its life. The best that can be made of the trouble of blindness is that it can be coped with, tolerated, and accommodated.[1] Accommodation and coping practices assume the form of medical, rehabilitative, and educational remedies designed to provide blind persons with various techniques required to cope with their blindness.

The trouble that blindness introduces into a life requires thought, and this thought is mechanical[2] in that it thinks only about the production of techniques for alleviating the trouble. The trouble with blindness is that it results, like any other trouble, in pain that must be eliminated by the production of techniques resulting from treating the problem in a mechanical way. Techniques such as orientation and mobility, and various kinds of technology, do alleviate to some degree the pain and trouble that blindness brings. But they do not rid the world of the problem of blindness.

Whether we are blind or not, a mechanical and technical response to life is necessary. Things such as telephones, computers, and automobiles are an essential part of our lives. This technology does remove the trouble of communicating over long distances, of storing vast amounts of

1   'Accommodation' is the contemporary way of speaking about disability, especially in the workplace. It is a legalistic term insofar as it springs from human rights legislation. Organizations are legally committed to providing disabled persons with the technical devices necessary for them to do their jobs. There is nothing wrong with this – nothing wrong unless this version of accommodation is the *only* notion of social relations that goes into achieving interaction with disabled persons. There is nothing wrong with this unless this version of accommodation prevents disability from influencing a workplace. This technical version of accommodation typically yields and makes possible disabled persons doing the same things non-disabled persons do and saying the same things, that is, 'fitting in' to a workplace not interested in difference, innovation, or vitality.

Zola (1982) speaks about the notion of technical accommodation – a notion that is pervasive throughout his work. He says that even though a workplace or any other location may be 'accessible' to disabled persons, it may not be welcoming. Accessibility, although necessary for participation, is not sufficient. This suggests that disabled persons are provided only with the *necessities* of life. But, to live a 'good life,' more than the provision of necessities is required.

2   For a discussion on the various distinctions of thought, see Heidegger, especially his *Discourse on Thinking* (1966) and his *What Is Called Thinking* (1968).

information, and of getting from place to place quickly. But, this technology does not address what it means to communicate, nor does it address the nature of a world that comes to value information as knowledge, and it does not address the nature of the need to travel. *Techne* is only part of the whole picture; it represents ways and means of conducting a life, but it does not represent the necessity of thinking about the value that makes it possible to conduct a life, any life. Blindness understood as trouble is only a part, albeit a necessary part, of the wholeness that is blindness.

But why is it so tempting to think of blindness only in a mechanical and technical way? Why is it so tempting to only develop techniques for either preventing blindness or coping with it? If *techne* is only part of the story, what discourages us from hearing or telling the rest of the story? What is it about blindness that makes us focus solely on the troublesome and technical part of its story? Is it that we do not know the whole story? Is it that *techne* is the whole story? Or, is it that the story of blindness is so nightmarish that we do not want to hear it? Nunez certainly wanted to escape from the country of the blind even if he had to die doing so. The person reading to Jenny could only 'blink' in the face of blindness. He did not want to hear the story Jenny's blindness was telling. Jenny was only beginning to learn that she had a story to tell.

Even if we do not know the story, we do know that one exists. And, even though we focus on the technical part of our life, we know that our life is more than the technical means we have invented for living it. Let us look at the nightmare that blindness, conceived solely as trouble, generates and paradoxically hides.

Trouble treats blindness as though it can be beaten since it can be coped with and accommodated. Nothing more has to be said or thought. The story of blindness ends here and remains untold. We can once more live in the 'sighted world' in a taken-for-granted way. The initial disruption to this world, and the resulting anxiety, can be put to rest by technically eliminating the trouble.

But it is precisely this anxiety, the anxiety of losing the security of the 'sighted world,' which gives rise to both thinking of blindness as trouble and taking technical steps as a way to remove the trouble. About such anxiety, Schutz (1973, 228) says:

... we want to state that the whole system of relevances which governs us within the natural attitude is founded upon the basic experience of each of us: I know that I shall die and I fear to die. This basic experience we suggest calling the fundamental anxiety. It is the primordial anticipation from which all the others originate.

From the fundamental anxiety spring the many interrelated systems of hopes and fears, of wants and satisfactions, of chances and risks which incite man within the natural attitude to attempt the mastery of the world, to overcome obstacles, to draft projects, and to realize them.

From the fundamental anxiety of death springs all other anxieties. It is this anxiety that generates our need to master the world. A need to master the world implies the fear that, if not mastered, it will master us. What does it mean to have the world as our master? What sort of master is the world? Surely, the world is, in part, the master we call nature. Modernity sees nature as an amoral and a democratic force, or better, a fair and just actor. Nature delivers her bounty upon us without regard for good or evil. And, without such regard, nature also delivers her wrath. Nature is fair and just insofar as she indiscriminately delivers what she has. Whether we are good or evil, rich or poor, white or black, men or women, she at one time delivers bounty and at another wrath.

We can now begin to understand the need to master nature. Any fair, democratic, or indiscriminate actor can be trusted to treat all of us equally. Such an actor gives no one any advantage. The actor who claims fairness as the animus of her action guarantees no favouritism. Whether nature delivers bounty or wrath, she claims no favourites. If we receive more wrath than do others, the rationale of nature is the rationale of accident, misfortune, and the like. The question Why me? is answered with a simple 'No reason.' This is why Kushner (1981) can write a book entitled *When Bad Things Happen to Good People.* Bad things do happen to good people, and good things do happen to bad people. There is no reason for this. We need not ask why; we need only ask what to do when good or bad things happen. The question What to do? is one way of avoiding the issue of developing an account[3] of our misfortune; it is a method for avoiding any thought about the idea that our master may have something in mind for us or that our master may be oriented in her action and may be acting justly rather than fairly. The question Why me? is shoved to the side by the question What do I do now?

Now that nature has delivered me the wrath of blindness, the question becomes What do I do in order to cope? The philosophic question of *why*

---

3 Another way to understand this book is to read it as an account of blindness. My aim is to develop an account of blindness as opposed to stipulating it and asking what can be done. For another example of the development of an account of blindness and disability, see Blum 1982. Giving an account of blindness is another way of saying that blindness has a story which needs to be told.

is abandoned in favour of the practical and technical questions of *what* and *how*. Now that I am blind, I must orient to, and learn, coping techniques so that, together with Kushner, I can orient my life to the fact that a bad thing has happened to a good person.

The occurrence, and thus the possibility of blindness, or any other wrath that nature might deliver, leads all of us to desire mastery over the world. The fair and indiscriminate master cannot be relied upon to tell us why or, for that matter, when she will deliver bounty or wrath. This produces anxiety since wrath may strike us at any time and for no reason. We need to predict. We need to gain knowledge of this fair master. We need to know why and when she will strike even though she herself will not, indeed cannot, tell us. We need to determine the conditions under which her wrath will fall. We need science. We need technology. We need modernity. We need the age of reason. We need to be able to predict the actions of this heretofore unpredictable master. We need to master nature, to master the world. And, when our mastery fails us, we learn to do what we need to do in order to cope. We treat blindness, or any other wrath, as the accident and failure of our own mastery. The accident of nature has been replaced by the accident of science and technology, by the inherent accident of probability.

The fundamental anxiety, our death, references the world as natural and, as such, as limited and mortal. Human life is embodied, and that embodiment, our body, is mortal – it will die. Like the life of our body, our sight will not last forever. But science and technology can allow us to make our bodies and our sight last as long as possible. We embark on projects that will 'probably' allow us to live and see as long as possible. If our life or sight leaves us prematurely, we will call it an accident, a disease, and we will cope. We will understand this premature death as yet one more occasion to understand and predict the indiscriminate actions of the world and as one more occasion to develop our mastery over that world.

Death and blindness represent the impetus for creating both prevention-of-death and prevention-of-blindness programs. Blindness gives us the impetus to develop coping techniques and thus to show nature that she is not the master but rather the subject of our actions. We can predict her actions with a high degree of probability, and, when our predictions fail, we can still master her by coping with these failures. Nature's wrath undoubtedly releases an unbearable pain. But modernity, in particular science, can alleviate the pain that nature delivers. We suffer, but modernity allows us to remedy, through various techniques, the pain caused by that suffering. What modernity and science do not allow, however, is the examination of the suffering itself. Suffering causes pain and it is only the prevention of this pain or the coping with the pain that science allows us to address.

The nightmare that the rest of this story of blindness reveals is the horror of mortality. It is the horror and nightmare of being blind in a world that sees. What if I could not see? What would I do? Who would I be? How could I master the world? Did nature win? Is she truly the master? If so, what else does she have in store for me? What happens to this world that not only I but everyone else takes for granted? Is it also mortal? How can I, despite my blindness, maintain the life of the world taken for granted? I must cope. I must take the world for granted. The world does see. I am an accident. I must be repaired and I must repair myself. The world does not need repairing; it is not an accident. But I am. That I am an accident and that I must cope and develop techniques for doing so forces me not to think of the horror that would follow if I were to think of the mortality of the world taken for granted.

Our modern time treats blindness as a condition that is accidental, troublesome, painful, and even inconvenient. It is a condition which is unnatural in relation to the natural. As an unnatural condition, blindness is understood as an accident of nature, as a disease, and so on. Nature did not intend to create blindness: blindness is merely an exception to the rule of nature; it is an anomaly.

There is no doubt that the occurrence of blindness provokes thought. It most often provokes the technical thought of what we should do. It provokes thoughts of gratitude and sympathy: gratitude, insofar as blindness allows those of us who see to feel grateful that we can do so; and sympathy, insofar as blindness allows those of us who see to feel sorry for those of us who do not. These thoughts are necessary and helpful. It can be argued that the very impulse to help springs from these sorts of thoughts. As an exception to the rule of nature, it is natural to think of a blind person as someone who requires help to reduce the pain and trouble created by this condition.

But this sort of thought does not allow for the possibility of blind persons requiring help with *understanding* their condition since this way of thinking always-already brings with it the ideology that blindness is an exception to the rule of nature. The only thought that is provoked is the thought which thinks about what to do with an exception. This is why the modern story of blindness is always a story of the exceptional and why what is not exceptional is never devastated by what is. Nature is not devastated by the unnatural since the unnatural never signifies the demise of what is natural. The unnatural is merely an exception and, as such, can be naturally explained, lived and coped with. This conception of the world provokes the mechanical thought that blindness is a physiological anomaly that produces negative effects on those who are blind. Thinking about how to minimize these negative effects *naturally* follows. Despite the necessity of this sort of thought, it nevertheless evokes only part of the story of blindness insofar as the meaning of blindness is not considered. Questions such as Who chooses to be blind? or What kind of blind person should I be? are nonsensical to the natural way of thinking that nature provokes on each and every occasion of the occurrence of blindness.

Such questions would evoke the one raised by Arendt (1958),[4] namely, Who am I? or Who am I, now that I am blind? Whatever we say and do, how we choose to live, always represents an answer to the question Who am I? We can say that whatever blind persons say and do, how they choose to live, represents an answer to the question What is blindness? Bringing Karatheodoris back, we can say that how we relate to blindness, whether our own or the blindness of another, and how we think of blindness represent an answer to the same question.

These sorts of questions are answered in modern times under the auspices of nature and reason. Even though blindness causes trouble, it is, nonetheless, an exception to the rule of nature. Blindness is not essential; it is not essential to human life as a whole, and it is not essential to the life of a person in particular. What is essential, from this point of view, is the natural-state-of-affairs that we call personhood. This is why so many blind persons today say that they are persons 'who happen to be blind.' They say that they are persons first and blind second. They say that their blindness is only an exception to the rule of nature, and therefore their blindness is inessential. Blind persons today are not required to think about the rule of blindness but, instead, are encouraged to think about what naturally rules them, namely, the rules of nature and of personhood.

The modern cry, indeed, the modern plea, of blind persons is 'I am not different. I am the same as you. You must please treat me equally.'[5] The modern cry is 'I am not a blind person, I am a person who happens to be blind. All of us, including you who can see, have things that happen

4 See especially pages 175–247.
5 The postmodern cry is somewhat different. It is wrapped in the cloak of relativism. It cries, 'We are all different. This makes us the same. What you see and what I see are different, but their worth is the same.'

to us. All of us, including you, are exceptional. None of us, including you, is perfect, is nature. Let us all treat each other equally since we are all the imperfect embodiments of nature.' Being in the same boat, we need only accommodate one another. There is nothing essential about what happens to us since what happens only produces trouble, pain, and inconvenience. This sort of thinking does, following Sartre (1948), certainly retain the essence of personhood, but, at the same time, it also annihilates the essence of blindness. This sort of thinking relegates blindness to the realm of personhood insofar as each and every one of us, blind or not, is not perfect. Even though we, as persons, are natural, we are not nature. We all lack, and blindness is just one more lack. It provokes the same kind of thought that all of us, insofar as we are persons and therefore troubled by our lack, require. Blindness provokes mechanical thought. This thought deflects us from thinking about blindness and forces us to think about it as lack and how to cope with it. This thinking forces us to take action rather than to think. As Heidegger (1968, 4) says, 'Most thought-provoking is that we are still not thinking ...'

The stories of Nunez and of Jenny point out a different path. It is the path to 'understanding.' Understanding, says Arendt (1994, 308),

... is unending and therefore cannot produce final results. It is the specifically human way of being alive; for every single person needs to be reconciled to a world into which he was born a stranger and in which, to the extent of his distinct uniqueness, he always remains a stranger.

Both Nunez and Jenny are specifically human, and both find themselves immersed in a world within which they are strangers. Nunez finds the country of the blind to be a strange land, and Jenny finds the same in the country of the sighted. But they are also familiar with their respective countries in that both of these lands are populated with human beings. Nunez and Jenny are simultaneously estranged from and familiar with their respective countries. They both seek an understanding of these lands by trying to reconcile the strangeness with the familiarity of humanity. Through no lack of trying, neither of them finds final results. Understanding is a path which winds through their countries and which takes them on an unending journey.

Blindness is such a path. It is a story which never ends. It is a life of estranged familiarity. Understanding such a life is an unending pursuit of the reconciliation between estrangement and familiarity. I will now turn to the specifically human way we come to discover our blindness.

3

Discovery

Blindness is usually conceived, first of all, as a condition and, second, as a medical condition and, as such, is open to diagnosis. Blindness does have a physiological manifestation which makes diagnosis appropriate. But my interest lies in addressing the whole of the story of blindness of which medicine and diagnosis are only one part. Even if I were to begin this discussion with diagnosis, I would have to develop that discussion in such a way so as to influence it to reveal many other aspects of blindness.

Diagnosis presupposes the experience of something wrong. It is this experience that leads us to seek diagnosis. But 'something wrong' is discoverable only through the living of our lives. Our lived experience provides us with the discovery of something wrong. The experience of discovery, unlike diagnosis, allows for the development and rediscovery of blindness in relation to the self, to sight, and to looking and seeing.

The discovery of something wrong is often experienced as surprise or even shock. We want to know what *went* wrong and what *is* wrong. But there is nothing unusual about this. When we experience something as wrong, we experience it as something out of the ordinary. Something that should be one thing is now experienced as another. We look, we see. Now we look and do not see. Something is wrong. Diagnosis comes into play only after the discovery of 'something wrong.'

The experience of something wrong is presupposed not only by diagnosis but also by discovery. Something wrong is an experience that is tied to the usual-state-of-affairs. Things of the life-world go along as usual in the way in which we expect. Part of our expectation is that things may go wrong. The usual-state-of-affairs involves the usual business of predicting, anticipating, and controlling things going wrong. Part of our orientation to the usual-state-of-affairs is to approach it with a certain sense of caution. Despite our complete trust in the life-world, we recognize, at least at some level, its vulnerability. We recognize its vulnerability to accident, injury, sabotage, and even to death: we recognize mortality. It is in the face of the mortality of the life-world that caution is born.

Caution is an approach we take to our bodies. We do so since we assume that our bodies are natural and should be healthy. Health is part of the usual-state-of-affairs. Our bodies *owe* us a natural life and a subsequent natural death. As a corollary to this, we take precautions insofar as our debt to the body is paid in the form of taking care that its naturalness stays that way. In our time there is a definite movement to the purification of the body.[1] We exercise, diet, avoid smoking, and the like. Those who do not are often spoken of as irresponsible since they do not recognize their debt to their body.

We assume health and ability until we have signs to the contrary. We take our sight for granted until we *see* some sign of something wrong. I will now examine these *signs* to see how they and their reading are played out in the social fabric of everyday life.

I lay there on my bed crying a little, but only a little, which surprised me because I was quite worried. I couldn't see the blackboard for the last couple of days now. But today, today was really tough. A line-drive was hit right to me and I saw it and then I didn't see it! It hit me right on the cheek. That had never happened before. I couldn't believe it – I saw it then I didn't see it. Laying there I didn't know what was wrong. Remember, I was only nine years old.

I could hear my mother and my grandmother talking in the kitchen. They were speaking their first language but I could understand them. My grandmother said she was getting old and that she couldn't hear well anymore nor could she see well. She said that soon she would die. My body froze in fright. I thought, I really thought, that I was dying. What else could it be? It seems silly now, but I spent the next few days testing my hearing to make sure that it was holding up.[2]

1 I address this issue in detail in 'Natural Childbirth, Physical Fitness and Natural Foods: The Purification of the Body under Modern Conditions,' paper presented to the Society for Phenomenology and the Human Sciences, Toronto, 1988.
2 Rod Michalko, 'White as a Cane: Stories of Blindness,' unpublished manuscript, 1996.

This is a story about going blind. This is my story. This is what I remember. This is a story of something going wrong and a story of how that wrongness is given life through the recognition that a life must be lived within the paradoxical awareness of the necessity and desire of life itself. It is the story of the necessity of diagnosis (what is wrong) and the desire for discovery (being wrong). Without the experience of something wrong, there would be no need for diagnosis. I was no longer able to see the blackboard or line-drives. Something was wrong – wrong with me. But, what? This question is the first element of the experience of something wrong, which leads to the need for diagnosis.

Diagnosis raises the issue of qualification. Only one who is qualified can say what is wrong, can make diagnostic sense out of the nonsensical experience of something wrong. The qualified diagnostician is often us; we experience something wrong, and we ourselves often provide a diagnosis. For example, we are driving our car down the street. The engine stops running. Something is wrong. We glance at the fuel gauge and see that it is empty. We have diagnosed the problem: we are out of fuel. The banality of the example aside, we can all recognize that type of experience and that type of diagnosis. We do so by virtue of our membership in a culture and our everyday experience of trouble, diagnosis, and remedy. This everyday 'trouble-diagnosis-remedy' algebra is an assumed quality of any adult member of a culture. The absence of such a quality often acts as a resource for jokes. 'Did you hear about the guy who was trapped on an escalator for four hours when the electricity went off?' Or, we all laugh at the person who, upon finding the lamp not working, calls an electrician, who finds the trouble to be a burnt out light-bulb.

But experiences of not seeing the blackboard or not seeing a line-drive are foreign to the language of the everyday trouble-diagnosis-remedy algebra. In that we experience something wrong, we do speak the everyday language of trouble. But when it comes to diagnosis and remedy, we are speechless. We turn to those whom we understand as qualified to speak the language of diagnosis and remedy; we turn to those who can tell us what is wrong and how to make it right again.

There are various versions of qualification. My grandmother possessed such qualification, though it was not steeped in her diagnostic powers as a medical practitioner but was born of experience. She was experiencing what I was experiencing. She was not seeing well anymore and neither was I. But what she possessed that I did not was an explanation; for her, the experience of not seeing well was the function of growing old, which, in turn, reminded her of her mortality. Lacking any other explanation, I did, at least temporarily, accept hers. I accepted her diagnosis, namely, that what was wrong with my eyes may be caused by my pending, not to mention premature, death.

The experiences of something wrong and of discovery are inexorably tied. Through my experience of something wrong, I had as a nine-year-old *discovered* the limits and the vulnerability of the body and, at least at some superficial level, the idea of mortality. No longer did I take seeing for granted. Until then, 'looking and seeing' was something that I assumed to be natural and unshakeable. I had discovered the fragility of that naturalness – of that looking and of that seeing.

Discovery comes to us wrapped within the mysterious cloak of serendipity. It almost seems to possess or, perhaps be possessed by, the unintentional character of accident, and it also seems, at least at first blush, to come to us without any trace of motivation.

The world appears to us to be different. We no longer see the world in the way we once did. What appeared before, now disappears. What we saw before, we no longer see. We do not experience this change in perception as located in the world itself. The world did not change. We did. What has changed is our *seeing* and not the seen *world*. The world is 'just there,' just there for us to see if only we were able to do so. 'Just there to see' always presupposes the faculty of sight and the capacity to see.

Discovering otherwise, we begin to mistrust the taken-for-granted character of sight and seeing. Bonner (1997, 84), making use of the work of Littlejohn (1989) and following Nietzsche, says that 'the discovery mode therefore requires that we treat any and all claims to truth with suspicion. This is the "art of mistrust" ...' This usage of 'discovery' leads to science. My usage is somewhat different. First, I do not treat discovery as a mode, and, second, the idea of 'mistrust' is not a requirement of discovery. On the contrary, discovery requires *trust* insofar as we trust the world to be what it is, and it is only the experience of 'something wrong' that leads us to make discoveries. The discovery of blindness requires trusting the reality of the world and its visual accessibility.

In his work on art, Gombrich (1960, 296) says that '... it is our knowledge of the visible world that lies at the root of all the difficulties of art. If we could only manage to forget it all, the problem of painting would become easy ...' Gombrich is referring to the work of other art theorists and argues against their understanding of the difficulty of the visual world. And, so he should. Forgetting that we know the visible world is an impossibility. At best, wanting to forget this is a complaint, on the part of artists, in the face of the difficulty in depicting the world artistically. This depiction involves *discovering* that visible world. Like art, blindness too wants to forget. But, like the artist, the blind person cannot do so. The artist and the blind person must confront the difficulty of discovering both their world and their depiction of it. The so-called art of mistrust is the mistrust of our depiction of our life in the midst of a world known and trusted. It is never 'easy' to capture the world artistically or to live in the world without seeing.

Unless we are artists or blind persons, seeing is easy. We typically do not distinguish between the sight we have and the sights we see; seeing these sights is good enough. We are satisfied with seeing whatever there is to see. Despite the ugliness of some sights, it is satisfying and even comforting to see them. Much of what we see today, we have seen yesterday. We are satisfied with this, and we are comforted that the world is what it is. The satisfaction and comfort of seeing resides in the pleasure of sensuality.

The sensuality of focusing our sight on a particular object or scene achieves the satisfaction of self-capacity. Resting our eyes blinkingly on nothing in particular achieves a kind of sensual pleasure that comes from trusting our eyes to see what they will and trusting that their will is unshakeably loyal to our will. Our eyes will see what they will until they perceive the desire of our will to see something other. Our eyes will see what they will until we desire to look. The sensuality of seeing resides in the notion that our sight can see and that our sight genuinely acts as a partner committed to the desire of our look.

Such a partner, a partner committed to our desire, is essentially playful. This playfulness is that of a lover. It is the playfulness of a lover who loves to see that at which the beloved wills to look. What seeing desires is our desire to look. The desire of seeing finds satisfaction in playfully inspiring us to look.

Even though the sense of sight is taken for granted, the sense of seeing is better captured within the web of the intermingling of desire and will. There resides in our body an intersubjectivity upon which all others draw (Merleau-Ponty 1968, 140–2). This intersubjectivity is between the subject 'I' and the subject 'eye' and the orientation that both have to each other in relation to desire and will. The one – I – desires to look, while the other – eye – desires to see.

Looking requires a subject in that it is necessarily steeped in decision. We *decide* to look at something by deciding to *notice* something that we are seeing. Our eyes see within, what is called by many disciplines from ophthalmology to philosophy, a 'visual field.' Our eyes see an entire field. Our eyes see everything there is to see but do not look at or notice everything they see. In contrast, our 'I' does not see everything there is to see, but it does look at everything it wills to notice. The intersubjectivity of the two consists in the relation between the desire to see everything and the will to look at something.

Deciding to look at or notice something is an essentially social act. Looking and noticing is located within the social web of interests, purposes, hopes, fears, anxieties, and so on. We are steeped in the life of a social world, with its scenes and events, which reveals itself to us only when we reveal our decisiveness to it. The revelations of the life-world are self-revelations. What we choose to look at reveals as much about us as it does about that at which we look. Our 'field of vision' is one way to speak of *how* the vast field of the social world becomes accessible to us. Seeing is one way to understand our need for accessibility to the social world. Looking and noticing are ways we have to speak about our need for participation in that world. Thus the relation between seeing and looking can be reformulated as the relation between accessibility and participation. It is our desire for participation that makes necessary our need for accessibility, and, in turn, the desire of accessibility is ultimately participation. We can only look at that which we can see; that is, we can only participate in that which is accessible to us.

The intersubjectivity of the 'I' and the 'eye' is a playful one, and this is what leads to discovery. It is often said that our eyes play tricks on us. We often notice things that are not there. The quintessential example of this is the mirage. We notice something that is simply not there. It is as though our eyes provide the noticeable thing (make it accessible) because our eyes understand our desire for noticing that particular thing. Our eyes can make us notice water when we are excessively thirsty; they can make us notice a friend when we are excessively lonely; they can make us see a dangerous person when we are excessively afraid; and the like.

'Seeing things' can be understood as our eyes' way of teaching us about excess. Our eyes have something to teach us about the excess of our need for survival and the excess of our emotional needs. Our eyes teach us about excess when they make accessible that which we want rather than that which we need. Our eyes teach us that we ought to address fear, loneliness, and even our bodily needs such as thirst. Through trickery, our eyes teach us to look at our interests. They teach us that *we*, and not they, are responsible for whatever it is we are noticing. It is as though our eyes love to see what we look at and will use trickery to remind us that such a love can be tainted by excess.

A version of the value of eyesight is the provision of accessibility. With-out it, participation is impossible. Our participation in the world is reliant upon accessibility to it. This is the value of eyesight. For most, eyesight represents the quintessential way of gaining access to the world.

The value of eyesight is born of the desire for participation. Its value lies in its capacity to make accessible various regions of physicality and sociality to our participation. When we lose our eyesight, we lose the valu-able accessibility to participation. This is the common-sense conception of the value of sight.

But this version of the value of sight is not a straightforward means/ends relationship. Accessibility and participation do not correspond to means and ends. Participation is not merely an end since it is more an on-going reachieving of human existence. Eyesight is not simply a means. It is not the instrument of accessibility. Instead, eyesight and accessibility refers to what things *should* be like. Being human implies access to the world. People should have access to it. This is part of the natural-state-of-affairs of humanity. Participation in the world presupposes accessibility not simply as a means but as an essential part of the human condition.

But when we conceive of accessibility and participation as a means/ends relation, we can very easily become obsessed with accessibility.[3] Means/ends thinking places accessibility and participation in a spatial relation. Accessibility comes first, participation second. Without accessi-bility there is no participation. Participation conceived as a concrete end requires the *a priori* of accessibility.

When eyesight is understood as the quintessential solution to the prob-lem of participation, blindness becomes the ultimate form of inaccessibil-ity. The blind person is understood as lacking, and what is lacking is the capacity *of* accessibility. The means/ends conception of accessibility and participation firmly roots the phenomenon of seeing within the experien-tial realm of the taken-for-granted. Participation is pervasive and is omni-present and co-present to all of us. We see people looking at all sorts of things: at television, at newspapers, at traffic lights, at each other, at them-selves. Such seeing presupposes that televisions, newspapers, or traffic

---

3 Accessibility is treated technically insofar as the assumption is made that persons with disabilities can be part of the world if care is taken to make that world accessible with remedies such as talking elevators, wheelchair ramps, and the rest. Much of the work produced in this area makes use of the rhetoric of 'accommodation' since it does not address participation. Participation presupposes accessibility but does not necessarily have a commitment to it. See, for example, Shapiro 1993, Weiner and Gallagher 1986, and Kunc 1981.

lights are accessible to those doing the looking. This is comforting. We are satisfied. Things *are* as they ought to *be*. The world is just there. It is just there because we can see that it is so. Thus, we can look at that world and participate in it.

Seeing and looking are a sense experience that allows for the sensual experience of moving freely through the world. Eyesight re-presents our desire to look at what we will. Our looking is a look of desire. Like a lover, the sense of sight fulfils our desire; it fulfils our desire for looking. Eyesight seduces us into thinking that all we desire to look at springs only from what is just there to see. We are seduced into thinking that our desire to look can only be satisfied by the sense of sight.

Thus blindness can only be conceived of and experienced as loss. The onset of blindness means that the taken-for-granted world can no longer be taken as such. Blindness also means that our desire to look at something which was at one time so natural is now so, so very, unnatural. Finally, blindness means that our looking is at a loss without the seductive lover of seeing. Discovery, wrapped in the experience of the something-wrong, represents this loss. This loss is experienced as a radical disturbance to capacity both in a kinaesthetic and social sense. It disturbs the stability of freedom that springs from the ongoing achievement of participation in a world. Discovering blindness in the experience of the something-wrong always precedes any diagnosis of it.

This is what a fifty-two-year-old salesperson, Nick, said of his initial experience of sight loss:

Well, ah, it was, it was really bizarre. I just finished a deal and I was on my way home. It was about seven o'clock at night and it was, ah, already pretty dark. Everything was going fine, it was only a ten mile drive. I pulled out onto the highway and, ah, after about a mile it starts going crazy. Everything went sorta orange or red or something. It sort of started slowly, but got worse and worse. Pretty soon, I could barely see anything. I remember thinking that this was the craziest fog I had ever seen. I remember getting home, but, to this day, I don't know how I did it. The biggest shock was walking in my front door. Then I knew, then I knew it was no fog. That's when, ah, that's when I found out later that my blood vessels burst.

Something was wrong, but, initially at least, what was wrong was a crazy kind of fog, which meant nothing was wrong with Nick's eyes. Nothing, that is, until he reached his home. It was then, and only then, that he discovered something was wrong with his eyes. Later in the interview, he told me that when he entered his front door and found everything inside to be orange as well, he was 'really scared.' 'I opened the door, walked in and just froze. Everything was orange, I couldn't believe it, I got really scared.'

Nick was scared and understandably so. He discovered in a dramatic way that it was not the fog that prevented him from seeing. His eyes prevented him from doing so. The source of the trouble was within himself and not fog. Entering his home was the point at which Nick discovered his blindness. The trouble which was outside came inside with him, and it did so because the trouble was Nick himself. It was then that Nick knew the world was clear, but that his 'seeing it' was not.

Initially Nick gave the benefit of the doubt to his eyes. Nick attributed his experience of something-wrong to fog. Strange as it might seem, and even though Nick thought it was a crazy fog, he did not lose trust in his eyes, in his seeing. His eyes had not failed him for fifty-two years, whereas the environment had fogged up from time to time. Fog was not only part of Nick's world but was also part of everyone's world. Nick trusted both the world and his seeing. He saw his world and saw that it was foggy. He saw a foggy world and *knew* that he was having trouble looking through it.

Until Nick entered his home that night, his trust in the world and in his seeing remained unshakeable. Nick followed himself home that night as much as the fog did. He saw something wrong. He saw fog. He assumed that the fog would end when he entered his front door. But what he saw followed him in. Nick froze because he saw fog inside. He looked inside and *saw* that he was not seeing. There was nothing to look at but the fog of not seeing. Nick could only look at his own *not seeing*. This is what scared him.

Nick saw his capacity for looking diminishing before his very eyes. Despite his desire for looking and his will to look, he could not. When he initially saw the fog, Nick thought that he was seeing merely one of the many sights the world offers. For Nick, there was fog and insofar as he saw it he knew he could see. But when the fog entered his home, Nick dramatically realized that he was not seeing. The fog was not one of the many sights of the world. In fact, the fog prevented Nick from looking at those sights. This is what scared him.

Later Nick received a diagnosis. The blood vessels in his eyes had burst, causing the orange-red fog. The diagnosis told Nick what was wrong. Nick had discovered something-wrong and the diagnosis named it. The diagnosis rendered an otherwise bizarre and crazy situation reasonable. Naming may be understood as one method that reason has for claiming discoveries. To name, to identify, to diagnose a thing, in this case a discovery, is to render it reasonable under the auspices of knowing and knowledge. Naming and diagnosing claim to know the thing that is wrong and thus claim the thing for themselves. Nick's lived experience of blindness remains his, but the name of his blindness is claimed by ophthalmology.

Ophthalmology can tell Nick more about his blindness than Nick can tell. Nick has the 'life of blindness,' and because it is a life, Nick cannot predict what will come in the future. On the other hand, ophthalmology holds all the names of blindness and knows these names well enough to offer a prognosis.

Ophthalmology often offers its prognosis in terms of its interpretation of accessibility and participation. A mother of a three-year-old blind child told me of her visit to a paediatric ophthalmologist. She described this visit as a 'follow-up' visit. Two weeks prior, her son was diagnosed as blind. This is how she recalled part of her follow-up visit:

It was sort of funny. He [the ophthalmologist] just sat there telling me about what Jamie's life would be like. He said that Jamie would be blind all of his life and there was like no cure. He said that there was nothing that could be done for him. Of course, I was feeling badly about this for quite a while now. But then he said something to me that made me feel even worse. He said that Jamie could never drive a car and he could never ski. Then he told me that Jamie would have to go to a special school for the blind and maybe he'd have to work in a special place for the blind. Then he said and like I didn't know what he meant here, but he said that Jamie probably couldn't get married.

Despite the extreme character of the ophthalmologist's prognosis, he was speaking in terms of accessibility and participation. The only prognosis the ophthalmologist made with reference to Jamie's blindness was that it would remain as diagnosed and that there was no cure and that it would be with Jamie for the rest of his life.

The prognosis said that much of the world was no longer accessible to Jamie and that this meant he would have extremely limited participation in that world. Driving and skiing were definitely out. Jamie would have to attend a special school, a school for students like him. He would probably have to work at a special place, a place for workers like him. And, he probably would not get married. Jamie could not look at what was necessary to look at in order to drive or ski. He could participate in school and in work, but only with like souls, only with those who also could not look.

Presumably, at least from this ophthalmologist's point of view, even marriage requires a sort of looking, a looking which the ophthalmologist understood as lacking in Jamie. (I will have more to say about this sort of 'looking' later.)

Jamie's mother was discovering cultural conceptions or collective representations of blindness. She was discovering what her culture has to say about its blind members. She was also discovering what her son would inevitably be discovering for himself as he grew older.

Jamie's mother told me that after that visit to the ophthalmologist, she felt worse and even a little afraid:

I actually was a little scared. I was scared for Jamie and what he would have to face. I didn't even know – I couldn't even think then how to help him. But then I thought, you know, maybe even I thought some of that same stuff that he [the ophthalmologist] did. After the first time, after he told me Jamie would be blind for life, I kind of thought some of that same stuff.

This is not necessarily guilt being expressed by a parent, nor only the expression of helplessness. It is the expression of membership in a collective that represents blindness in the negative form of lack. It is a collective that represents blindness in terms of what-cannot-be-done – in terms of an inaccessible world often hostile to and fearful of the idea of blindness. It is the fearful discovery of the power of representation. Jamie's mother discovered her own participation in a collective which was only now becoming accessible to her. Ironically, Jamie's blindness brought his mother's collective into view. She could now *look* at the collective she always saw. Jamie's blindness inspired his mother to look and fear that which she saw.

This sort of fear is not unusual. This is what a thirty-year-old man told me he remembered when he lost his sight through what was later diagnosed as retinitis pigmentosa:

My eyes kept getting worse. It really was like looking through a tunnel. And at night, well, I couldn't see a thing. At night I was total. But I remember when it first started happening, I thought, I thought, well, I couldn't do anything. But then I thought geez I'm gonna be a blind man. I thought, I really thought I'd have to sell pencils or something. Then I thought that everyone was looking at me and thinking I was just helpless. I didn't blame them, really, I thought I was helpless too. What can I do? No more going to hockey games. I won't even be able to play with my kids anymore.

This man, Bill, lost his sight in adulthood. And, unlike Jamie, Bill was already discovering and facing various conceptions of blindness. Despite their age difference, Bill and Jamie shared something in common. Blindness was *new* to both of them. Bill is concerned about 'who he is' now that he is a 'blind man.' Jamie has no such concern. But Jamie's mother certainly does, and she expresses this concern on Jamie's behalf.[4] Jamie and Bill share the same concern: they are both concerned – Bill on his own behalf and Jamie through his mother – with the question Who am I now that I am blind? However, Bill is an adult and Jamie is a child. This difference does not erase what Bill and Jamie have in common, but it does distinguish them with respect to how they relate to the question about who they are now that they are blind. Jamie's mother *knows* what Jamie will inevitably face, and Bill *knows* what he is already facing.

What Bill is already facing are representations of blindness that are present in his life. Blind persons *cannot* watch hockey games, they *cannot* play with children, they *cannot*... Blind persons are simply helpless. Bill has already discovered that he *cannot*... and Jamie will inevitably do the same. This is what provides for their simultaneous sameness and difference.

Bill already knows that blindness represents a loss. He knows this because he once possessed what is now lost. At one time, Bill could see whatever there was to see and decided to look at whatever he decided to look at. When Bill became a blind man, he lost the sensuality of seeing that satisfied and comforted his desire to look. Bill lost access to the life in which he participated, thereby losing access to his own life.

Losing one's sight is 'losing sight' of one's life. When Bill lost his sight, he lost access to his life in relation to his desire for participation. Bill was now a 'blind man.' He was a man without access to the world, which meant he was a man who was 'helpless.' At one time, Bill understood himself as not helpless. He *had* help – sight. Thus, Bill is an expression of the collective representation of blindness as needful of help. As a blind man, Bill needs help. The ultimate form of help that he needs is his sight.

Bill discovered his helplessness only when he discovered his blindness. He discovered the helpful character of his seeing only when he lost it. Bill lost the help he needed to satisfy his desire for participation. There is no longer any sense of comfort for Bill in relation to his participation in his life. He is no longer comfortable with the possibility of attending hockey

---

4 For an excellent discussion on the development of the need to speak on the behalf of self, see Blum and McHugh 1984, 239–45. These authors also explore this issue by making use of the work of Piaget (ibid., 123–42).

games or with playing with his children. In fact, the very idea of attending a hockey game or playing with his children makes Bill uncomfortable.

Bill is not saying that he literally could not attend a hockey game since he surely can. What he is saying is that there would be nothing comforting in this insofar as he could not *look* at the hockey game. Bill could 'be there' but does not see a way that he could participate. To be there is not the same as 'being there.'[5] Bill is saying that being there presupposes that the 'thereness' is accessible to being and accessible to whomever is there. This accessibility makes possible the claim to 'being there.'

There is something ingenuous, for Bill, about being somewhere without experiencing its thereness. Bill finds something discomforting in being a spectator at a hockey game without being able to see the spectacle. He is afraid that people will look at him. There is something discomforting in a spectator becoming a spectacle.

A young blind man once told me that he attended a striptease club with a friend who was sighted. One of the strippers noticed his white cane and thus him. The stripper then came to where they were seated and asked the young man's friend why he brought this blind man to a strip club. This young blind man became a spectacle instead of a spectator. Blindness always becomes a spectacle when it appears in an environment conceived as essentially visual.

Before he lost his sight, Bill attended hockey games. He was a spectator. But now that he is blind, Bill does not feel comfortable with himself as spectator. Any spectator without the qualification of sight is, for Bill, not only discomforting but ingenuous. Such discomfort and ingenuousness are often experienced in interactions between blind and sighted persons, especially when such interactions make use of visual metaphors. Sighted persons often feel uncomfortable and even embarrassed when they say things such as 'See you tomorrow' or 'See you later' to blind persons. There is often a sense of ingenuousness at play when a blind person says, 'I saw her yesterday' or 'Yes, I saw that movie.' In its literal sense, this sort of interaction makes the claim of being able to look at what there is to be seen. It is with this that Bill, now that he is blind, feels uncomfortable.

A blind woman, Gertrude DeLeo (Levine 1976, 23), puts the matter this way:

5 Kosinski (1970) dramatically illustrates this point. Chance, a most appropriate name, 'is there' insofar as he is perceived as participating in thoughtful reflections about the current state of America. However, Chance is there merely by chance. He himself is not participating. Chance is there without ever being there.

Unsighted people use the words: look, see, I see you. We're trying to sound as much like our seeing peers as we can. It is looking in our sense. The thing is that we don't want to constantly remind someone that we are blind. I think that's true in terms of me in any case. I'd like them to think in terms of talking along with their friends. To think of me as one of them, not a blind person. And if you are going to say, may I feel that, then immediately the person realizes. But you can catch them off guard and you can say, may I see it. It's just the desire to be one of the sighted world. I think it's an anxiety to a degree. It's one of our many anxieties, but of course all of us have anxieties.

This sort of reasoning implies a descriptive fidelity in phrases such as 'May I see that' or 'See you later' when used by sighted persons. Sighted persons can actually look at the thing they ask to see, and they can actually see you later. This descriptive fidelity cannot be attributed to these phrases when used by a blind person. They cannot look at things the way sighted persons can nor can they see anyone later, or now, for that matter.

Such usage represents, for DeLeo, a desire to be 'one of the sighted world.' It represents the desire for participation. It is her way of looking, her way of participating. To speak of a 'sighted world' or of 'sighted peers' is to express the desire for participation in relation to the need for a world-in-common. Through language, DeLeo not only represents her desire for participation but also depicts one method for its achievement and hopes to depict her blindness as secondary to her personhood.[6] She takes care that her desire for participation (e.g., talking with people) will not 'remind' those with whom she is talking that she is blind. DeLeo does not want anyone to 'look' at blindness when they 'see' her. She will not ask to 'feel that' since that sort of usage will make her interlocutors mind-full of her blindness. She does this in hopes of reminding others that blindness is part and not the whole of who she is.

DeLeo does recognize that using such phrases as 'May I see it' may catch sighted persons 'off guard' and does recognize that such usage is fraught with anxiety. There is almost a pathos that springs from the recognition of the distinction between the world of sighted persons and the world of, to use DeLeo's term, the 'unsighted.' DeLeo's reflections are

---

6 Sartre (1948) speaks of this issue within the paradigm of 'democracy.' Democracy suggests equality insofar as all of us should be treated equally despite our differences. Sartre suggests that one method for doing so is the evocation of the notion of 'personhood.' This means that we can all depend on the fact that we are 'persons' as a way to remove any difference that may exist between ourselves and others. I can always count on the fact that I am a person as a way to diminish the influence of the fact that I am blind.

the beginning of the distinction between *how* sighted persons look and see and *how* blind persons 'look and see.'

This demarcation represents a development in discovery beyond that made by Bill. Bill's discovery of blindness distinguishes blindness from sightedness in relation to participation; sightedness is participation, whereas blindness is not. DeLeo develops this distinction in her discovery that, despite the distinction, both blind and sighted persons desire participation. Despite the anxiety and pathos, DeLeo will do what she *will* in order to represent that desire as indistinguishable. Her interaction with sighted persons is animated by a desire to *remind* sighted persons that, like sightedness, blindness too is *deeply* needful of participation.

Despite individual differences, there is something common to all discoveries of blindness. Everyone discovers their blindness as a life lived in the midst of both sight and sights. This inevitably leads to the discovery of the *tragic* conception that the life of sight and sights *ought* to be lived by those who are themselves sighted and can see. The discovery of blindness makes us mindful of the 'better life' of seeing and thus of the hegemony of the senses in relation to perception, accessibility, and participation.

Discovering blindness is the discovery of tragedy. Tragedy often helps form the discovery of blindness. This is particularly true in the case of congenitally blind persons. Their discovery of blindness is certainly different from that of adventitiously blind persons. Kevin, blind from birth, told me:

I'm not sure how old I was. I guess, I guess it was quite young because it was long before I went to school. I must have been around two or three probably. Anyway, I remember that the girls upstairs were playing something. They were laughing and everything. I wanted to join them so I went upstairs and asked them if I could play. They laughed even harder. I remember that they were quite firm. 'No, you can't play, you have to see to play this game.' I didn't even know what they were talking about. But I do remember that I knew, for the first time, that I was different somehow.

Like all two- or three-year-olds, Kevin does not know about himself. We must all discover that we are boys or girls, that we are rich or poor, that we are black or white, and so on. We must also discover that we see or not. Being born blind or sighted does not in and of itself provide for the understanding that we *are* blind or sighted. This must be discovered and it must be discovered through the living of a life.

Kevin began his discovery of blindness through the tragedy of exclusion. But he was not excluded on the basis of race or gender. He began the discovery of *his* difference through the discovery of inability and incapacity. Kevin could not play, not because he was a boy, but rather because he could not see. He could not play because he *could not play.*

Kevin's story of his discovery of blindness is accompanied by the discovery of inability. This is true even for DeLeo, who has been blind for many years and has known of her blindness for many years. Still even she is reminded, particularly when she interacts with 'sighted people,' that a blind person cannot 'see that' or cannot 'See you later.' Even DeLeo is reminded of the possibility that sighted persons may discover inability when they discover blindness. She is aware that her participation in the 'sighted world' provides for the possibility of her being interpreted as someone who is incapacitated. She is aware that she may be interpreted as someone whose participation is limited in a way that the participation of sighted persons is not.

This awareness *may* be the source of some of the many anxieties of which DeLeo speaks. Perhaps DeLeo is anxious about the risky character of interaction and the particular risk that the introduction of blindness brings. She does suggest that she does not want to interact in a way that would remind persons of her blindness. She says that using the phrase 'May I feel that?' instead of 'May I see that?' would be a clear reminder of her blindness.

However, DeLeo uses a dog guide. Since a dog guide signifies blindness, DeLeo is not interested in 'passing'[7] as a sighted person. Whatever else a dog guide means, it does not mean that the person using it is attempting to 'hide' her or his blindness. DeLeo is not trying to hide her blindness by using phrases such as 'May I see that?' or 'See you later.' Presumably, her dog guide reminds people that DeLeo is blind.

We cannot take DeLeo literally when she says that she does not want to remind sighted persons that she is blind. DeLeo must have something else in mind when she says this. DeLeo's blindness is obvious both to herself and to others. There is thus something other than blindness of which DeLeo does not want to remind others. It is inability that DeLeo wants to keep out of the minds of others. She does not want to live the life that embodies inability. She does not want anyone to discover inability when they discover her. DeLeo's desire, one fraught with anxiety, is to be one of the many participants in the 'sighted world.' DeLeo is explicitly concerned with depicting her ability to participate.

7 'Passing' is explored fully in chapter 5.

It is the potential failure of such a depiction that makes DeLeo anxious. Saying 'Let me feel that' or 'Let me see that' are both risky. The one reminds others of inability, while the other catches them 'off guard.' This makes DeLeo anxious. She is anxious about her participation in a world and is ultimately anxious about the living of her life. DeLeo joins all of us, those of us who see and those of us who do not, in the essential anxiety and risk of living our lives. But for DeLeo, and perhaps for many of us, this is still to be discovered.

Diagnosis remains hidden in the murkiness of the discovery of blindness. Nevertheless, it does have a place in the story of blindness. What part does diagnosis play in this story? Parents of a blind child said:

Okay. She was 3½ months old when we noticed that she wasn't following objects. And, I guess because she was our first child, we didn't really realize that she should have been seeing much earlier. Nothing, nothing. Well, her eyes were jumping ... And we had an impression that she was looking at things. I guess what she was doing, she was just ... her eyes were so close to your face when she was looking at things. And it turned out that she wasn't really. That was just an impression.

So, you did notice the eyes ...

They were jumping ... We noticed that ... moving ... Yeah. A lot of jumping around ... unsteady ... flickering ...

So, what did you do? Did you say ...?

No. Nothing at the time because, uh, I don't know ... We had read about it or people had told us that it's quite normal, apparently it is, quite normal that immediately after birth a baby's eyes can, often, do jump around and do all kinds of things. Because, in fact, in retrospect, when we talked to the, our paediatrician and mentioned this, you know, this whole problem that people had said babies will often do this, he said, yes, as a matter of fact that he did notice the flickering and he wrote it off as being the same thing. Oh, yeah, that's not a serious thing. That's quite often how it happens. It goes away. Well, it didn't really go away entirely ... We started ... well, actually we started suspecting that she wasn't going to walk into the room and, rather than looking over at you which by that age we thought that she should, she just kept, maybe, looking up at the ceiling or whatever, or at something else. So, then we started ... Paediatrician, yeah. And then he referred us to a neurologist who works with the eye. He was hoping that it was another problem rather than blindness, I think.

How do you mean he was hoping that? Did he tell you that?

Well, he probably thought it was a brain problem or something. Or something that can be operated on. Something other than blindness. I guess he didn't want to frighten us. And then, once the neurologist gave his version, then we would look into the eyesight, because he basically had told us after his examination that there is a problem. That was our biggest shock. This was before we went to the paediatrician. Once we noticed that she wasn't, you know when we walked into the room, like I mentioned before, didn't look at us or hand us something, the odd time, I don't know; you have something in your hand and you thought that she should be looking at it ... Anyway, when we started suspecting that there might be something then we went into her at say, night-time, when she was lying in her crib and just took in a flashlight. And started to fool around with the flashlight and we basically got the same reaction as what the neurologist did.

This brings us full circle. We began this chapter with a discussion of the relationship between discovery and diagnosis. I spoke of discovery as the finding of 'something-wrong' and of diagnosis as the finding of 'what-was-wrong.' The comments of these parents will assist in understanding this relationship better.

These parents have discovered something wrong in the way that their daughter was looking and seeing. They wonder whether or not their daughter *could* look and see. Their daughter's eyes moved, jumped, and flickered. She did not appear to look at anyone or at things that she should have seen. Something was wrong.

Because they were first-time parents, they did not possess the experience that would tell them whether something was wrong or whether this experience was merely a part of normal physiological development. They had heard and read that these sort of signs often occur in children and are often corrected through normal development. Even though the parents had discovered something wrong, they were not sure whether something was *really* wrong or not. They were not certain what it was they had discovered.

Thus the parents conducted tests. Interestingly enough, the tests they conducted were similar to those conducted by their doctor. Their 'flashlight test' told them that their discovery was, *in fact*, a discovery of something wrong. They knew that they had discovered something wrong with the way their daughter was looking and seeing.

It was then that the parents decided to consult those who are qualified and expert in the ways of looking and seeing. They consulted the disciplines of paediatric ophthalmology and neurology, and eventually they did receive a diagnosis. 'At the end, they told us that she was blind and that she would be blind for the rest of her life. You know, we sorta knew that. But we were still really shocked.'

Even though these parents 'sorta' knew what was wrong, they 'checked.' They checked with parents, friends, books, their obstetrician, and ultimately with the flashlight test. Finally, they checked the validity of their diagnosis with a neurologist. They checked their experience as well as what they made of that experience.

Checking the validity of experience is certainly not something peculiar to these parents. All of us conduct such 'experience checks,' especially when we experience something out of the ordinary. Experiencing something out of the ordinary is what generates the 'double take' or, the more contemporary, 'reality check.' Without the out-of-ordinary experience, emotions such as surprise and shock would be impossible. We live our lives with the tacit expectation of a certain order of things. We expect that our life will unfold in the way that lives generally do. Disruption to such an unfolding is what yields the out-of-ordinary experience, which, in turn, yields the checking of such experiences as a method for accepting them or not.

The checking of extraordinary experience is not confined to the experience of something-wrong. We also check extraordinarily good experiences. For example, we 'pinch ourselves' when we win the lottery. We hope that we are not dreaming. The same rationale holds when we try to confirm our discovery that there is something wrong with our child's eyes. We hope that we are having a nightmare. All checking of out-of-ordinary experience is done under the auspices of hope.

All discoveries bring with them the need for hope. We hope that our discoveries will turn out good and not bad. In the case of particularly shocking discoveries, we hope that we are having a nightmare and are not awake. And with particularly good or surprising discoveries, we hope that we are awake and not dreaming. Thus we check our experiences. Diagnosis enters the picture with hope as well. We seek a diagnosis with the hope of discovering the nature of our discoveries.

Hope connects discovery and diagnosis. Discovery is the experience of finding, and diagnosis is the experience of thinking about or *theorizing* it. The experience of discovery is often fraught with passion (surprise, shock), whereas reason (calculation, rationality) often animates diagnosis. Discovery and diagnosis represent the voices of passion and reason that play together and struggle with one another in the arena that we call 'our life.' It is the voice of hope that mediates the conversation between passion and reason. We can hope that our passions, our experiences, will be thought about and reflected upon, and we can also hope that our reflections will be embellished by passion. Our discovery of our blindness, together with its diagnosis, can *hopefully* free the voices of passion and reason so that we may discover something about *our self.*

Diagnosis has provided us with the opportunity to discover the need to theorize our experience. And, diagnosis is one form of such theorizing. Even though diagnosis leads only to a treatment of blindness as a condition, its aim is to understand blindness.

Diagnosis introduces another voice in the story of blindness. This voice is represented in the disciplines of rehabilitation and special education. Ophthalmology's aim is to diagnose and treat blindness. Thus its voice speaks of blindness as a condition amenable to such treatment. But this is where ophthalmology ends. It turns the conversation of blindness over to rehabilitation.

That rehabilitation speaks next is no accident. Its voice is oriented. Rehabilitation will enter the story of blindness only after ophthalmology is through speaking. Both disciplines understand this. Rehabilitation will not speak until ophthalmology gives it permission to do so. Both are committed to blindness and both have something to say about it. However, these two voices never interrupt one another. Rehabilitation speaks *because* ophthalmology is done. From this point, ophthalmology remains silent and contributes nothing more to the story of blindness.

Rehabilitation and ophthalmology possess a mutual understanding in regard to who speaks when in the story of blindness. Ophthalmology, as a sub-discipline of medicine, is a significant voice in this story, but its significance is short-lived. This itself is significant. Medicine suddenly relinquishes its voice to rehabilitation. It is worthwhile examining the significance of this sudden relinquishing of a voice.

Medicine has a great deal to say about blindness; more than anyone else, it knows about the physiology of the eyes; it knows how eyes *ideally* work and why they do not. Medicine knows why people are blind. It organizes this knowledge through the development of a taxonomy of eye conditions. It can tell us what eye conditions obtain, along with the nature of such conditions, that together act to produce blindness. Medicine has much to say about blindness and, in this sense, is extremely vocal. But suddenly, it falls silent. It has nothing more to say, and, even when asked, it refers all queries to rehabilitation.

Perhaps the answer to the question of ophthalmology's silence in regard to blindness lies at the heart of medicine itself. The diagnosis of incurable blindness means that it is not possible to restore sight. There is no cure. From a medical point of view, blindness is a physiological condition that, like any other such condition, is subject to the medical ideal of cure. It is the possibility of cure that permits medicine to remain in the conversation of blindness. Curative action is medicine's only recourse to discourse after diagnosis.

The impossibility of a cure renders medicine hopeless. Where there is no hope, medicine bows out. This cure/hope dichotomy has existed in medicine, at least in terms of Western civilization, since the time of Hippocrates:

Giving up a hopeless case could be justified by the Hippocratic rule that it was an essential part of the medical art 'not to take in hand those overpowered by the disease.' Shortly before his death, and despairing of the political situation in Rome, Cicero wrote to a friend, 'Hippocrates too forbids employing medicine in hopeless [cases].' (Temkin 1991, 139)[8]

What is clear in this passage is medicine's commitment to cure. The content of the passage, namely, that medicine ought not deal with hopeless cases, is possible only when the notion of cure is presupposed. It is this commitment to cure that makes it possible and even necessary for medicine to consider at least some cases hopeless.

Hippocrates, generally thought of as the parent of contemporary Western medicine, recommends that medicine, then considered an art, ought not take 'in hand' those who are 'overpowered' by disease. Medicine, now a science, has a sense of the potentially overpowering character of disease. Medicine's fundamental commitment is to do everything in its power to overpower disease – to cure. It takes disease in hand until it becomes overpowering, and then it is out of medicine's hands. The one afflicted with an overpowering disease has no other choice but to *wait*, and to conceivably die doing so, for medicine to find a cure, thus regaining its power. In the case of incurable blindness, the blind person has no other choice but to *live* with blindness, cope with it, adjust to it; the blind person has no other choice but to *wait* for ophthalmology to find a cure.[9]

Medicine does not consider living with the disease as having it 'in hand.' For medicine, living with blindness resembles more Vladamir's waiting for Godot than it does the life of Zorba's dancing. Blind persons

8 Hippocrates (1978, 67) developed an 'oath' for medicine, which in part reads: 'I will use my power to help the sick to the best of my ability and judgement; I will abstain from harming or wronging any man by it.'

9 People living with AIDS make a similar argument in relation to the medical conception of AIDS. See, for example, Gott 1994.

do not dance with their blindness; they do not embrace it. Instead, they wait with their blindness; they cope with it and adjust to it.

It is this idea of waiting as much as it is the idea of hopelessness that *makes* ophthalmology bow out of the conversation that constitutes the story of blindness. What do any of us have to say to someone who is waiting? At worst, we chit chat, we pass the time of day. At best, we talk about that for which they are waiting and how well they are coping with and adjusting to the wait. Waiting for something is not typically conceived as being as enjoyable as having the thing itself. We are often impressed by those whom we think of as waiting well. We are impressed with those who wait patiently or who are courageous in their waiting or who find humour in waiting. We are impressed with a 'spirited' wait. Ophthalmologists are impressed with blind persons who cope with or adjust to blindness. Medicine may be impressed with the power of those who wait patiently in the face of an overpowering disease.

Ophthalmology treats blind persons in a way that resembles Beckett's characters who spend their lives waiting for Godot. Beckett's characters often say, 'Nothing can be done,' nothing, that is, except waiting. Ophthalmologists often use a similar phrase when they tell people that their blindness is permanent or incurable. They often say, 'Nothing can be done.' Incurable blindness means that there is nothing more to do and nothing more to say. There is nothing that ophthalmology can do or say that will change permanent and incurable blindness into sight. Like Hippocrates, ophthalmology recognizes hopeless cases, and, like him, ophthalmology sees no point in taking these cases in hand.

Thus ophthalmology falls silent in the face of blindness. It cannot do what it does. In hopeless cases, it cannot restore sight. Again, like Hippocrates, ophthalmology characterizes as 'hopeless' those cases it diagnoses as incurable. What is hopeless is the 'case.' 'Case' is a medical gloss insofar as that term glosses over what is meant when it is used. Using the term presupposes an understanding of the meaning to which its use points.

From ophthalmology's point of view, hopelessness explicitly points to, in Hippocratic terms, disease. Certain diseases, specifically those which are overpowering, do not respond to the curative measures of medicine. No matter what medicine does, these diseases continue. It is as though they do not subject themselves to the 'doings' of medicine. Medicine deems these diseases hopeless.

But there is another aspect to the hopeless case. Disease is *always* made manifest and expressed *in* a person. People make it possible for disease to come alive. Thus medicine treats 'diseased people' and not disease. Medicine treats people with disease. The criticism that medicine often treats only the disease without considering the person notwithstanding, it can treat nothing other than a person. This criticism refers to the bureaucratic way that medicine often carries out its treatment. It refers to how medicine often treats disease without respect for the person who has the disease. Whether medicine respects the person or not, it cannot deny the fact that disease is always expressed in a person.

An overpowering disease overpowers both the person and medicine. The power of a person and the power of medicine are no match for the power of some diseases. Hence, hopeless case.

But the gloss 'hopeless case' is also used by medicine, albeit implicitly, to preserve the power of the person. A person with an incurable disease is indeed powerless but only in relation to the disease. The person is powerless only when characterized as a 'hopeless case.' Ironically, the gloss 'hopeless case' holds out hope for the person. This hope resides in the understanding that medicine 'hopes' that the diseased person possesses the power to live with his or her disease in a spirited way. Medicine hopes that persons with terminal illness, for example, will evoke a 'will to survive,' and it hopes that persons with a permanent medical condition such as blindness will evoke the 'will to adjust.' While medicine holds out no hope for hopeless cases, it holds out hope for the person.

This paradox generates particular responses from medicine. Individual medical practitioners are characterized by some as compassionate or dispassionate, as friendly or bureaucratic, as responsible or irresponsible. Medicine is often criticized when its response is directed *only* to the case in exclusion of the person. These are the dispassionate, bureaucratic, and irresponsible practitioners. Those practitioners who direct their attention to both the person and the case are conceived as compassionate, friendly, and responsible. Thus practitioners may respond either bureaucratically or compassionately to the paradox of hopelessness and hope.

'Guilt' is another response of medicine. Blindness is often surrounded by guilt. Parents often feel guilty when they produce a blind offspring; blind persons themselves often feel guilt for their own blindness; sighted persons often feel guilty in their relations with blind persons; and so on. This sense of guilt is no foreigner to medicine.

A mother whose daughter was blinded shortly after birth puts the matter of guilt this way:

They were supposed to check her the week before she was to go home. And, for some reason, the guy missed her that week and caught her the next. Donna was the worst case they'd had in five years, the only really definite blindness case they had had in five years. I think they were just as upset as we were. They were even more upset because at one point they said, 'Oh oh, I don't know how you can even talk to us.' I said, 'Well I wouldn't even have her if it wasn't for you.' They felt so guilty. Oh, they really felt awful.[10]

Donna's birth was difficult for two reasons: first, she required incubator treatment, primarily for the provision of oxygen; and, second, the excessive oxygen caused retinal damage that led to her blindness.

Even though Donna's mother expressed gratitude to them, the hospital staff felt awful and guilty. These feelings were generated by a sense of negligence. The medical staff were *supposed* to check Donna and for some reason did not. In fact, they did not check Donna until the week after she was scheduled to be checked.

The medical staff saved Donna's life. Yet, they felt guilty. Guilt came with the diagnosis of blindness. They had made a mistake and missed the scheduled check that would determine whether Donna's retinas were reacting negatively to the provision of oxygen. Prudent action may have avoided blindness.

Had Donna not 'gone blind,' there would have been no guilt. The medical staff surely would have received a scare and even felt relief that the missed check had not resulted in any tragedy. But as for feeling awful or guilty, no, of course not. The presence of blindness, the presence of a medical tragedy, the presence of a negative medical consequence, these are the conditions for the onset of guilt. The diagnosis of blindness brings with it the need for a 'cause.' Any medical diagnosis ideally includes the source (cause) of the diagnosed condition. In Donna's case, the source was medical negligence. The guilt that surrounds blindness was doubly felt by the medical staff since the source of the diagnosis was their own administrative 'snafu' – situation normal all fouled up. Not only was normal medical practice fouled up, but Donna's normally seeing eyes were also fouled up.

This double dose of guilt was made even clearer by the attending paediatric ophthalmologist. Soon after Donna was diagnosed as blind, the paediatric ophthalmologist spoke with Donna's mother and told her, 'What's even worse is that there is nothing we can do about her blindness, it's permanent. I'm really very sorry.' The ophthalmologist said that *we*

10 It is interesting to note that this mother is also a nurse. Perhaps her involvement in the medical profession accounts, in part, for her forgiving attitude.

cannot do anything about Donna's blindness. The 'we' signifies the discipline of ophthalmology. *Ophthalmology* can do nothing about Donna's blindness. But then, 'I'm really very sorry,' says the ophthalmologist. As a person, the ophthalmologist is sorry that Donna's blindness is 'permanent,' meaning that she is sorry that Donna will have to live with blindness for the rest of her life. As an ophthalmologist, her apology is also spoken on behalf of the discipline. The ophthalmologist is sorry, 'really very sorry,' that her discipline cannot do anything about Donna's blindness. There is nothing more that ophthalmology or the ophthalmologist can do about Donna's blindness since 'nothing can be done.' However, the ophthalmologist did tell Donna's mother that she could 'refer them to the CNIB' (Canadian National Institute for the Blind).

Ophthalmology's *raison d'être* is, following Hippocrates, to conserve and to restore sight. Not doing so represents failure. Failure sometimes generates guilt, so much so that some ophthalmologists seek professional therapeutic help. Cholden was one of the first psychiatrists to document this phenomenon; he (1958: 22, 24) puts the matter this way:

... the doctor who in his daily work devotes himself to the conservation of sight often reacts emotionally to its loss ... there are a number of reasons for this. Blindness may be seen by the doctor as a failure of his own ability, or as a loss of his self-esteem, or as an injury to his reputation ... for the doctor to tell the patient with finality that he is blind might be conceived of as a reflection both on the power of the doctor and on the power of medicine. It indicates the limit of the physician, and who among us wants to know our limits?

First, we learn that doctors may react emotionally to sight loss. Second, we learn that blindness may be seen by the ophthalmologist as a failure of his/her abilities or loss of self-esteem or even as an injury to reputation. Finally, we learn that blindness may be interpreted by ophthalmologists as a reflection on the power of an ophthalmologist and on medicine. Blindness may indicate the limits of ophthalmologist and ophthalmology.

From this, we get a much clearer understanding of why ophthalmology falls silent regarding blindness after its diagnosis. Speaking in this situation invokes the possibility of failure, of loss of self-esteem, of injury to reputation, and of limits. If ophthalmology continues to speak about blindness after its diagnosis as incurable, it may be asked to account for its limits. As Cholden says, '... who among us wants to know our limits?'

There are many of us who want to know our limits. But this is not my point. Rather, my point is fixed on the pursuit for the grounds of ophthalmology's silence in the face of blindness.

As a discipline whose commitment is the conservation of sight and as practitioners who accept the responsibility of carrying out this commitment, ophthalmology and ophthalmologists face the possibility of hopeless cases. They approach their work with some understanding of the possibility of failure. Ophthalmology knows that it will not be able to conserve the sight of everyone who sees; thus the need for on-going research. Ophthalmologists know that their practices and procedures will not always be successful. Both know that they will, from time to time, confront cases of overpowering blindness. On this issue, a retina specialist admitted the following to me:

We know a lot about the retina and generally our treatments are very successful. But there's still lots we don't know. We're still battling with RP and macular degeneration. Sound treatment for these sorts of problems is still a ways down the road. Our research is getting close though.

The use of the pronoun 'we,' together with terms such as 'treatment' and 'research,' suggests that this ophthalmologist is speaking on his own behalf and on behalf of his discipline. Both are successful and both face hopeless cases. Even though ophthalmologists know that their practices and procedures will sometimes be unsuccessful and even though they know that their discipline must continue to conduct research as a consequence, they still react emotionally to failure. The same ophthalmologist also said:

I don't know, it still makes me feel bad. Every time I get a case of RP, I know I can't do anything about it. There is just no treatment. They're referred to me and they come in here hoping, just hoping, I can help them. And, you know, I can't. The only good thing, if there is anything good here, is that I can refer them to the CNIB. You know, rehabilitation can help them and then there is all kinds of technology nowadays.

At least, nowadays, there is rehabilitation, which alleviates, at least somewhat, the pain of the ophthalmologist. Unlike Hippocrates, who was without the profession of rehabilitation and would not take hopeless cases 'in hand,' the modern practitioner has somewhere to 'hand' his or her hopeless cases. However, both amount to the same thing: not taking hopeless cases 'in hand' or 'handing' them to some other discipline means, essentially, that medicine can do nothing else and has nothing more to say.

The last utterance comes in the form of the pronouncement of a hopeless case. Other than saying it is incurable, ophthalmology has nothing more to say about incurable blindness.

Yet, some ophthalmologists feel badly about making such pronouncements. As Cholden says, sight loss often leads to ophthalmologists' reacting emotionally, losing self-esteem, experiencing injury to reputation, and the like. Blindness often brings ophthalmologists face to face not only with the particular limits of their practices and procedures but also with the limits of their discipline. Blindness represents a disruption to medicine's commitment to the conservation of sight. Blindness disrupts the 'aim' of ophthalmology.

Aristotle says, 'Every art and every inquiry, and similarly every action and choice, is thought to aim at some good; and for this reason the good has rightly been declared to be that at which all things aim' (Aristotle, *Nichomachean Ethics*, 1094a1). If all things do aim at the 'good,' then ophthalmology must do the same. If every art, inquiry, action, and even decision (choice) also aims at the 'good,' then ophthalmology, certainly a form of inquiry, certainly action, certainly decisive, and possibly even an art, must also do the same. What, then, is this good at which ophthalmology aims? 'Healthy eyes' comes immediately to mind. But Aristotle distinguishes between the 'end' of action and the 'good' toward which it aims. He says that health is the end of the art of medicine (ibid.). Thus, 'healthy eyes' may be more the 'end' of ophthalmology than the 'good' toward which it aims. The good of ophthalmology resides in the accomplished end of healthy eyes. The good of ophthalmology is understood from the standpoint of whether or not it is successful in achieving its end. As Aristotle suggests (ibid.), the end is more important than the action; in this case, the end of healthy eyes is more important than the practice of ophthalmology. Whatever ophthalmology *is*, it is secondary to its end of healthy eyes.

But healthy eyes as an end is the same as ophthalmology insofar as healthy eyes mark both ophthalmology's end as well as the end of ophthalmology. If everything, including an end, aims at some good, then we must look elsewhere to *glimpse* the good toward which ophthalmology aims. Ophthalmology can tell us whether or not our eyes are healthy, and it can sometimes correct our unhealthy eyes. But it would be a mistake to conceive the good of ophthalmology as its end of healthy eyes. Such a mistake is precisely what leads ophthalmology to react emotionally to the failure of its practice. When ophthalmology equates its standard for its action as the end of healthy eyes, it necessarily *deeply* fails when it *concretely* fails to live up to its standard. When the end of healthy eyes is the *only* standard to which ophthalmology is obliged, its success or failure depends solely upon whether or not it achieves this end. Failure is restricted *only* to ophthalmology. All things we are involved in sometimes fail and at other times succeed.

We often react emotionally to failure. Ophthalmologists are no different. They involve themselves in the 'thingness' of ophthalmology, and sometimes it fails. Thus, guilt. Guilt is part of the 'gestalt' of ophthalmology. Failure, like ophthalmological practices and ends, is but a part of the whole of ophthalmology. Failure is a derivative of the practice and end of ophthalmology.

It is precisely in this sense that blindness acts to remind ophthalmologists of their limits. Blindness reminds ophthalmology of the limiting character of its practices and of its end. Its practices often fail and so too do healthy eyes. There is a limit, or mortality, to healthy eyes insofar as, with age, they often grow weak or, at some point, simply fail. There is a similar limit to ophthalmology insofar as its practices often fail or its theory sometimes cannot account for certain eye conditions.

But to return to our question: what 'good' does ophthalmology, with its practices, its theories, its failures, its successes, to what 'good' does it aim? We must turn our attention away from ophthalmology *per se* and focus more on the end of ophthalmology. We need to look more closely at 'healthy eyes' as an end. It is this end upon which ophthalmology hinges its esteem and reputation. What does ophthalmology hold in the *highest* esteem? There must be something that ophthalmology values even more than itself, something that would, in turn, provide not only for the possibility of ophthalmology but also for its self-esteem. Ophthalmology could not have generated itself, and thus it must find its generation in something other than itself. Ophthalmology *must* have an origin.

The end of healthy eyes must have some particular significance for ophthalmology. But this significance is not self-evident. The only thing that is self-evident is whether or not eyes are healthy. For example, obstetricians can see healthy eyes in a newborn. They can also detect unhealthy eyes. Obstetricians can detect, for example, congenital cataracts in a newborn through the observation of excessive cloudiness in the newborn's eyes. The medical 'gaze'[11] can see healthy eyes. However, the significance and value of this observation are not themselves observable.

---

11 Foucault (1973) speaks of the medical gaze as part of his work on the 'archaeology of medical perception.' Phrases such as 'see a doctor' or 'be seen by a doctor' do not signify anything visual, at least, in common-sense terms. Instead, such phrases make reference to the *way* medicine sees as opposed to the way other interests do.

Since the significance and value of healthy eyes are not an empirical matter insofar as they are not directly observable, they must be tacitly brought to that 'gaze' which empirically observes healthy eyes. The value that generates the desire and need to empirically observe eyes as a means to detect either their healthy or unhealthy character *must* necessarily precede any empirical observation. The value of healthy eyes itself marks the origin of both the condition of healthy eyes and the need to observe that condition.

'Healthy eyes' signifies some *necessary condition* to some value. We all know that the condition of healthy eyes means that we can see. (The opposite is also the case.) The ability to see means that we are able to fulfil the desire to look. It means also that we can live sensually with the sensuality of the world. The 'gift of sight' presents us with the highly esteemed gift of 'opportunity.' The significance and value of healthy eyes amount to the gift of accessibility to a sensual world represented in the opportunity to participate in that world.

The condition of healthy eyes represents the opportunity to live a 'life of sight' – a life *lived* with sight and sights. Healthy eyes signify the *opportunity* to 'be there visually' in a world that offers itself through sights. Healthy eyes signify life itself. This is no different from the condition of birth since both represent the 'value of life.'

From ophthalmology's point of view, the ability to see is inexorably tied to this value of life. It is this value which represents the 'good' toward which ophthalmology aims. There is no value, for ophthalmology, in the condition of unhealthy eyes since they do not signify accessibility and thus do not represent the opportunity for participation. This is the pathos of the hopeless case.

The observation of either healthy eyes or a newborn bears the imagined potentiality and possibility framed within the value of opportunity. The newborn represents the imagined life to be lived. It is not 'looked at' merely as physiology. Instead, it is looked at as gender, as race, as class, as hope, as embodying the 'chance' to decisively live a life. Nor are healthy eyes 'looked at' merely as physiology. They are looked at as having will and sensuality, as being revealing, and as possessing the ability and the chance to fulfil the decisive desire to 'look.' Healthy eyes and the newborn are the same insofar as they both represent the opportunity for participation in the world and the chance that participation will be decisively influential on the world. This means the opportunity of the newborn is also another chance not merely for survival but for a life that has not been lived before. The opportunity of healthy eyes represents the chance not to merely look and see what there is to be seen, but to look and see what has never been seen before.

For ophthalmology, blindness is hopeless. It is hopeless because when it is observed there is no imagined opportunity. Instead, blindness is imagined as *the sense of lack* – that shadowy sixth sense. The blind person has no opportunity to look at what there is to be seen. Neither does he or she have the chance to see what has never been seen before. This is why ophthalmology reacts emotionally. It sees hopelessness when it looks at blindness and is hopeless in this looking.

And this is precisely why ophthalmology turns to the disciplines of rehabilitation and special education. These disciplines act as a backstop for ophthalmology, somewhere for it to throw (refer) its hopeless cases. For ophthalmology, rehabilitation and education represent hope. They represent the hope that at least some opportunity, limited as it might be, can be provided to the blind person. Ophthalmology can provide no chance for blind persons and understands that their only chance lies in the arenas of rehabilitation and education. From this point forward, ophthalmology falls silent. Although it no longer speaks, ophthalmology does listen. It listens for hope in the story of blindness and turns its ear to rehabilitation in the hope that the silence will be broken.

4

Rehabilitation

The stillness that befalls the story of blindness is short-lived. Breaking the stillness is the voice of rehabilitation. Despite its silence, ophthalmology prepares the way for rehabilitation to enter this conversation, to become a storyteller. It does so through the 'referral.'

Following a diagnosis of incurable blindness, ophthalmology refers the case to rehabilitation. Ophthalmology still responds to questions insofar as they are framed within a language that both enables and empowers it to speak. Here, for example, is what a young man asked his ophthalmologist after a diagnosis of incurable blindness. 'Do you think, is it possible, that I can get some other eye problem?' To this his ophthalmologist replied, 'That's possible. But that's why you should come back for checkups on a regular basis.'

Note that the ophthalmologist does not continue to speak about the young man's permanent blindness since he has nothing more to say about it. Yet he does have something to say about the question posed to him. The ophthalmologist's response could have been a response to any one of his patients. Any patient may ask questions regarding the possibility of future 'eye problems.' It is no surprise that the ophthalmologist responds to the young man's question. The young man asks about the possibility of any *other* eye condition, and his question is not directed, and does not direct the ophthalmologist, to the eye condition that is responsible for the onset of his blindness. The question acts to alert the ophthalmologist to ignore the current eye condition. It gives the ophthalmologist permission to respond *as if* he was speaking only of future eye problems. The question gives the ophthalmologist a way to speak ophthalmologically.

In contrast, other sorts of questions render ophthalmology silent and elicit responses that are preparatory. After receiving the news that she was permanently blind, a thirteen-year-old girl asked her ophthalmologist, 'But what, what do I do now? I mean do I, I mean can I keep going to school?' Her ophthalmologist responded, 'There are all sorts of things. There are many ways to keep going to school. Actually, I'll refer you to the CNIB. In fact, I'll speak to your parents about it in just a minute.' This girl's question does not give her ophthalmologist permission to speak ophthalmologically. Her ophthalmologist has nothing more to say. The girl's question permits the ophthalmologist to speak *only* within the framework of preparation. His response prepares the girl and her parents for what he and his discipline do with hopeless cases. The ophthalmologist has begun the process of handing over a case that is no longer in his hands. The ophthalmologist is making a referral. He is telling the girl that he is done with her and is done with her story. Her particular story of blindness, steeped as it is in her life, will now have to be told without any further responses by, or any further conversation with, her ophthalmologist. The referral is ophthalmology's method for bowing out as storyteller in the story of blindness and is its way to introduce the next speaker.

The ophthalmological referral to a rehabilitation agency such as the CNIB brings with it the notion of recommendation. Ophthalmology *recommends* rehabilitation as the 'next step' in the development of blindness. It conceives of rehabilitation as the quintessential solution to the problem of permanent blindness.

It is in this sense that the referral resonates with recommendation. Recommendation is, following Wittgenstein (1958, 168e, ff), part of the 'grammar' of referral. In the *speaking* of referral, we unleash its language, which reveals recommendation as fundamental. When we speak a referral, we are, simultaneously, recommending that to which we refer. When ophthalmology refers a blind person to a rehabilitation agency, it is recommending both that agency and the practice of rehabilitation. Ophthalmology is recommending *agency* as an *actor* presented as qualified to speak about, and act upon, permanent blindness. This suggests that blindness requires agency and needs to be acted upon in order for it to be lived with.

To rehabilitate (*re-habilis*, or *rehabilitatio*), according to the *Oxford English Dictionary*, is 'to restore to former status.' We see that rehabilitation is committed to some 'former status' and to the value of 'restoring' that status. This commitment reveals the beginnings of a conception of blindness. Rehabilitation must conceive of blindness as a status needful of restoration. Blindness is a status born out of a former status. As a status needful of restoration, blindness must be connected to a former status; that is, blindness must have originated in some different, but connected, status.

Rehabilitation conceives of the origin of blindness as located in something *other* than itself. Blindness is not original insofar as it is conceived as both subject to, and a subject of, restoration. Restoring blindness to its former status is restoring it to what it originally was, namely, sight. Like ophthalmology, the end of the former status to which rehabilitation is committed is sight. Rehabilitation, too, conceives of the seeing life as the only good life.

The trouble here is that it is difficult to understand how rehabilitation can actually restore sight or even be committed to that end. We have no difficulty in understanding that ophthalmology's commitment is ultimately sight restoration. We can also understand why ophthalmology celebrates its successes in this endeavour and laments its failures. But in the case of rehabilitation, understanding this is not so easy. Not only do we not easily understand how rehabilitation can celebrate success in its attempts to restore sight or lament its failures, we do not easily understand how rehabilitation can be committed to sight restoration in the first place. Yet, rehabilitation is committed to restoring blindness to its former status. Since the status that blindness formerly held was sight, rehabilitation is committed to nothing other than the restoration of sight.

The commitment to restoring something to its former status suggests that the thing to be restored is itself of no value in its current status. We can begin to understand how something conceived as needful of restoration is itself a thing thought about as a 'mere shadow' of its former self. Blindness becomes a mere shadow of its former status. The metaphor 'shadow' has two meanings. First, anything seen as a mere shadow of its former self is understood as less than or not as good as the original. There is a quantitative and qualitative difference between the self and its shadow. In the quantitative sense, a person who loses a significant amount of weight, for example, is often characterized as a mere shadow of his or her former self. The qualitative sense of shadow is often characterized in terms of the comparison of ability. Mere days before his retirement and after several knee operations, the great Bobby Orr was reported to have said, 'Skill-wise, I'm only a shadow of what I used to be.'

The second meaning that shadow comes with is that of image. Images suggest distortion and they are ever changing. For example, at one time a shadow is long and at another, short. A shadow follows something 'real' and clings to that reality for its life. No 'real thing' can ever rid itself of its shadow. This means that any reality, or any version thereof, casts a shadow of itself. Reality, regardless of how it is conceived or how it is spoken of, casts shadows, and thus images are part of any conception of reality. To the extent that they are part of reality, shadows are often confused with, and mistaken for, the thing that casts them. As Plato describes in his metaphor of the cave (*Republic*, book 7), many see only shadows when they look and are thus satisfied with the life that does not look at all there is to be seen. Many see images as all there is to see, thus looking at only part of reality and thereby mistaking the part for the whole.

The rehabilitative conception that blindness is a mere shadow of its former self suggests that blindness is a shadow of sight. Rehabilitation sees blindness as a shadow but does not see sight as such. Blindness shadows sight, clinging to it for its existence yet never managing to be anything more than sight's mere shadow. Rehabilitation sees sight as a real thing and not, therefore, as a shadow or image of anything. Sight *is* status and is a status *former* to blindness. Sight is not a mere shadow of its former self since it has no former self. Thus sight is not regarded as needful of restoration. Only the ever-changing and distorted character of shadows and images needs to be restored to the unchanging clarity of their former status. Unless an image is returned, through restoration, to the origin of which it is a shadow, it will always remain a mere shadow of its former self. In this sense, rehabilitation is committed to restoring blindness to its former status (sight) and thus returning it to its rightful origin.

But there is more to rehabilitation:

Rehabilitate – 1a. to restore by formal act or declaration (a person degraded or attainted) to former privileges, rank, possessions; to re-establish by authoritative pronouncement. b. to re-establish the character or reputation of a person or thing. 2. To restore to a previous condition; to set up again in proper condition. (*OED*)

The latter part of this definition gives a version of rehabilitation's conception of shadows and images. They are incomplete, distorted, and defective in relation to their origin. It is in this sense that rehabilitation can speak of itself as committed to the restoration of a 'previous condition' or the restoration of a 'proper condition.'

We can begin to glimpse the *moral* character of rehabilitation. It is committed to 'previous' conditions which are 'proper.' In our earlier example of weight loss, we can understand how someone who was previously obese would not be committed to restoring this current condition to the previous one of obesity and would certainly not see obesity as the proper condition. What was restored was the original condition of a healthy body.

Sight restoration is a method 'to set up again in proper condition.' Blindness is understood as an improper current condition in relation to the previous and proper condition of sight. Thus rehabilitation sees sight as the proper condition. It is a condition that each and every one of us *should* 'properly' possess. This is the moral character of rehabilitation. Everyone *should* see and everyone *deserves* to see. Therefore, rehabilitation *must* see a blind person as a person *whose sight is missing*. A blind person is a person who is missing the condition of sight, a condition which *properly* belongs to that person.

What, from this standpoint, do we see when we see a blind person? What do we see when we see a person whose sight is missing? What do we see when we see a person who *should* see and *deserves* to see? What we see when we see a blind person is a *sighted person* whose sight is *missing*.

It is from this point of view that the argument over whether it is better to have had something and lost it or better not to have had the thing at all, gains its relevance. Is it better to have sight and lose it than not to have had sight at all? is a question that often springs to mind, especially in the face of blindness. This sort of question gains its relevance from the notion of knowing or not knowing what we are missing. Is it better to know what we are missing or not? Whether or not we know *what* we are missing, we do know *that* we are missing it. Blind persons know that they are missing their sight. And, it is this knowledge that gives rise to the question of whether it is better to have had sight and lost it or not to have had it at all. Both sides of the argument presuppose that sight is missing.

We can begin to understand rehabilitation's commitment to 'declaration' and to 'pronouncement' as a method for re-establishing a person who is 'degraded or attainted'; for re-establishing a person's 'former privileges, rank, possessions' and 'the character or reputation of a person.' The fundamental interest of rehabilitation goes beyond the mere restoration of a previous condition. Rehabilitation is fundamentally interested in the restoration of a condition or status in which, before restoration, a person lives in degradation with an attaintment or, as Goffman (1963) might say, a 'stigma.' It is interested in restoring privilege, rank, possessions, character, and reputation. Living a life in the way it *should* be lived is rehabilitation's fundamental interest. Living a life without 'proper conditions' is not worth living.

With proper conditions as its end, rehabilitation embarks on its path of restoration. It 'declares' and 'pronounces' it. This sounds as though rehabilitation need only stipulate a life as restored. This may be understandable when it comes to restoring a person's privileges, rank, and possessions or even when it comes to restoring a person's character or reputation. We can understand, for example, a court of law restoring someone's privileges or possessions. Or, we can understand how someone's reputation can be vouched for as good by declaration or pronouncement. However, it is more difficult to understand how someone's sight can be restored in the same way.

Declaration and pronouncement bring with them the idea of 'authority.' These are signifiers of authority. Authority is required for declarations and pronouncements to be heard as such. Any declaration or pronouncement is authoritative and, in this sense, is a 'formal act.' They are acts that are 'authored' by the legitimacy that resides in the author.

In the case of sight restoration, ophthalmology is conventionally understood as the authoritative voice. Ophthalmology often 'declares' an eye condition as ophthalmologically treatable, thus rendering that condition restorable to its previous condition of sight. The eye condition is 'in hand,' and the ophthalmological (authoritative) pronouncement is that the proper condition of sight *will* be re-established. Ophthalmology acts, and does so formally, as the author of such a pronouncement regardless of which individual ophthalmologist utters it. In contrast, persons who lose their sight may receive pronouncements from their friends that their sight *will* be restored. But these sorts of pronouncements are spoken from the auspices of friendship and are thus heard, at best, as 'best wishes' or, at worst, as 'wishful thinking.' Friends may offer condolences and support to those who lose their sight. However, friendship does not offer the authority to pronounce a condition restorable. Ophthalmology can speak authoritatively about sight restoration, whereas friendship cannot.

The contrast between ophthalmology and friendship does help to point to the idea that ophthalmology is typically considered as the quintessential authority on sight restoration. Rehabilitation makes a similar claim. It claims that blindness is amenable to restoration and thus claims that the condition of blindness can be restored to its origin. To grasp this, we must first understand rehabilitation's conception that a blind person is a sighted person with the sight missing.

Selma Fraiberg, herself an educator of blind children and a researcher, commands tremendous respect within the education and rehabilitation community. In regard to the idea of 'missing' which I have been trying to address, she writes:

What we miss in the blind baby, apart from the eyes that do not see, is the vocabulary of signs and signals that provides the most elementary and vital sense of discourse long before words have meaning. (1977, 95–6)

We notice that Fraiberg uses the term 'miss' in a way that depicts two different meanings. First, the blind baby is born with something missing. Insofar as it is born with 'eyes that do not see,' it is born without seeing eyes, it is missing eyes that do see. Second, we, and I assume that by 'we' Fraiberg means sighted persons, 'miss' the baby's seeing eyes. But we do not miss them in the way the baby does. Instead, we miss the baby's seeing eyes in a dramatic sense, almost akin to the way in which we miss a friend or loved one who has died. A deceased friend or loved one is no longer here and will never again be here, and it is their 'hereness' that we miss. We miss their vitality and their discourse. We miss their life *here* with us.

For Fraiberg, we miss the seeing eyes of the blind baby in a fundamental way – we miss the most elementary and vital sense of discourse with the baby. We miss the ability to 'be here' with our baby in a discursive way that is most elementary and most vital. Missing such an ability is not something we find to be missing in ourselves. Eyes that see give people this ability. Thus they have the ability to engage in the most elementary and vital sense of discourse. The blind baby is missing this ability and we miss it.

The blind baby is missing a 'vocabulary' of 'signs and signals' that 'provides' for a fundamental discourse. If the baby was born blind, this vocabulary would not be missed since he or she would not have had it in the first place. It is we who miss this vocabulary.

Fraiberg draws a connection between eyes that do not see and the missing vocabulary. But she expresses this connection in an automatic way. It is as automatic a connection as the one that appears between genitalia and gender in a newborn. See a penis, see a male.[1] See eyes that do not see, see a missing vocabulary. This 'seeing' necessarily blurs the social character of the achievement of the connection between genitalia and gender as well as between eyes that do not see and a missing vocabulary. This seeing is itself blind to the social character of both gender and blindness. It is to the socially organized character of blindness that Scott (1969, 121) speaks when he says, 'Blind men are not born, they are made ...' Scott's analysis does point to the usually ignored idea that blindness is not mere physiology insofar as it encompasses the makings of social action

---

1 Bonner (1984) provides an analysis of this taken-for-granted connection in his work on birth announcements.

and interaction. It takes more than a penis to see a male, and more than eyes that do not see to see blindness.[2] This sight is missing in Fraiberg.

Fraiberg de-emphasizes the physiological aspect of blindness (eyes that do not see) in favour of emphasizing the social character of blindness, namely, a vocabulary of signs and signals. She is saying that the meaning of blindness can be addressed only when its physiology takes a back seat to its social character. This is the fundamental reason for ophthalmology handing the conversation of blindness over to rehabilitation.

Even though Fraiberg and hence rehabilitation speaks of the meaning of blindness as located in the web of social action and interaction, we need to look more closely at their viewpoint in order to discern their particular conception of the meaning of blindness. Fraiberg treats blindness as a phenomenon steeped in lack. What is lacking is the capacity for the 'most elementary and vital sense of discourse.' The blind baby is not able to enter into a discursive relation with adults, and presumably other babies, since it lacks that which signifies and signals the capacity to do so. This baby gives no sign or signal to others which would allow them to interpret him or her as either engaged, or potentially engaging, in discourse.

This sense of discourse, according to Fraiberg, comes 'long before words have meaning.' Presumably, a baby with eyes that do see possesses the capacity for such discourse long before it can utter meaningful words and long before it can understand the utterances of others. Still, this baby *must* possess some version of speech. The seeing baby communicates long before the spoken word has meaning.

This communication consists of the 'signs and signals' which make up a 'vocabulary.' We can imagine what Fraiberg means when she speaks of signs and signals; she means the 'non-verbal' vocabulary that most of us assume and take for granted as one of the features of a baby. She means things such as the movement of the baby's eyes which eventually leads to 'eye contact,' the movement of its hands and arms toward objects of interest, smiles, and the like. She means all the things that adults have come to expect babies do as part of their communicative repertoire. She means, finally, all those things that babies do that are read by adults as attentiveness, as interest, as 'normal' development, as satisfaction, as dissatisfaction, and the rest of the signs and signals that make up the vocabulary

2 This notion is not exclusive to blindness but pertains to other disabilities as well. Poitras Tucker (1995, 209), for example, writes, 'For thirty-six years I buried my deafness in a hole so deep no one ever found it, and I would not allow *myself* to find it.' Hearing deafness takes more than ears that work.

that babies have that, from the adult point of view, provides for their capacity to enter into discourse with adults in the most elementary and vital way.

But these signs and signals signify something else. This vocabulary is heard by adults as telling them that the baby is responding properly to sense stimuli. Adults hear this vocabulary as saying that the baby possesses the 'proper condition' that positions her or him in the status of a sensorial and sensual being. The vocabulary says that the baby has sense perception. The baby has senses that sense. The vocabulary says that the baby has eyes that *do* see; it says that the baby is sighted, and, more dramatically, it says that the baby is *not* blind.

Contrary to Fraiberg and rehabilitation, the absence of such a vocabulary in a baby also signifies and signals something. Such an absence signifies and signals that something is missing in the baby. Regardless of how this 'something' is interpreted, it is nonetheless communication; it is a vocabulary that provides for the most elementary and vital sense of discourse. This vocabulary, described by Fraiberg as 'missing,' tells adults just that; it tells adults that something is missing in the baby. Both the presence *and* the absence of a vocabulary of signs and signals in a baby are, in an elementary and vital sense, discursive.

Even though Fraiberg makes use of the vital discourse of blind babies, she ignores their discursive practices. The blind baby must have 'told' Fraiberg something in order for her to see that the baby is lacking signs and signals. The blind baby must have told her, in one way or another, that she or he does not have these signs and signals. The blind baby must have given Fraiberg *some* sign and *some* signal that he or she lacks those signs and signals. Ironically, both Fraiberg and rehabilitation suggest that blind babies tell them that they (the babies) are lacking a vocabulary of signs and signals, and they do so *with* the vocabulary they supposedly lack.

Fraiberg is simply wrong in her judgment of the communicative abilities of blind babies. Assuming that her error is not steeped in some limitation of intellect, we must look elsewhere for its source. We might even admit that our judgment that Fraiberg has committed an error may be a little strong and even somewhat premature. I say this not as a way to withdraw my initial judgment but, rather, as a way to come to an understanding of how blindness comes to be interpreted as well as to an understanding of collective representations of blindness which act so as to provide for various individual interpretations of what blindness is.

The work of Gadamer can assist in this understanding. In his discussion of the 'hermeneutic circle,' he says,

The circle, then, is not formal in nature, it is neither subjective nor objective, but describes understanding as the interplay of the movement of tradition and the movement of the interpreter. The anticipation of meaning that governs our understanding of a text [vocabulary of signs and signals] is not an act of subjectivity but proceeds from the communality that binds us to the tradition. (Gadamer 1975, 261)

The interpretation of what Gadamer calls a 'text' or, in our present case, the interpretation of the behaviour of a baby first as signs and signals, second as a vocabulary, and finally as the elementary and vital sense of discourse springs not from the subjectivity of a person (the interpreter) but rather from the relation (interplay) between a person and a tradition. No one approaches a phenomenon alone. We move through the world of phenomena with our interests, concerns, purposes, fears, hopes, and anxieties, as well as with our traditions.

Since we move through the world with our individual particularity together with a tradition, our interpretation of that world with its multitude of phenomena, including babies, necessarily expresses our subjectivity in a way that shows our commitment to a tradition. We are bound to a tradition insofar as it influences our individual particularity and thus influences how we 'see' and interpret the world. The reverse is also the case; hence the hermeneutic circle. How and what we see proceed from a community bound in the interplay of persons and tradition. This is why Fraiberg and rehabilitation belong together. Fraiberg's interpretation of blind babies does not spring from her individual subjectivity. Instead, it is an interpretation accomplished through the interplay between Fraiberg and the tradition of rehabilitation.

This interplay sheds some light on why Fraiberg ignores the presence of a vocabulary of signs and signals in a blind baby, while at the same time she relies on their presence for saying that they are missing. The tradition of rehabilitation provides a framework for seeing blindness as a lack. Thus Fraiberg is not merely interpreting blind babies. She is 'seeing' lack when she sees a blind baby and is interpreting this lack as requiring the intervention of sight. Fraiberg (1977, 283) says,

Finally, the effects of intervention can be summarized: In those cases of development where comparative data are available, our educationally advantaged blind infants came closer to sighted-child ranges than blind-child ranges.

At least one of the reasons for Fraiberg's ignoring a vocabulary of signs and signals in a blind baby is so clear now that it practically jumps out at us and seems too obvious even to address. Nevertheless, one of the commitments of the tradition of rehabilitation is to understand and interpret the behaviour of a baby as a vocabulary that provides for the most elementary and vital sense of discourse, a discourse which, in turn, signifies a baby's *development*. When rehabilitation *sees* a baby, it simultaneously *looks* at development. What a baby says to rehabilitation when the baby reaches out its arms, follows objects with its eyes, and the like is whether or not it is developing normally. Rehabilitation understands the baby as *decisively* saying this since what the baby is saying may be interpreted in other ways. Reaching hands, smiles, etc., may be read as affection, or as discomfort, or even as humour. Now it is true that even these attributes may be thought about in terms of development. We could say that a baby is developing a sense of humour. On the other hand, we could say simply that a baby *has* a sense of humour. However, Fraiberg's 'look' at a blind baby is a representation of her commitment and tie to the tradition of rehabilitation and its particular interest in the development of blind infants.

What is rehabilitation's interest in this development? What guides the look of rehabilitation to a baby? Babies are interesting. But our concern here is to explicate the particular kind of interestingness that babies acquire from the point of view of the tradition of rehabilitation.

Fraiberg has developed 'ranges' of development for both blind and sighted babies. Like the rest of us, Fraiberg and her tradition of rehabilitation see babies as developing beings – beings 'on-their-way-to-adulthood.' Thus babies are understood, not as persons, but as *potential* persons. Babies represent the potential for full-fledged, *bona fide*, and competent membership in society. It is in this sense that babies are seen as 'on-their-way-to-personhood.' Babies are interpreted within the paradigmatic schema of *potentiality*. As potential and as on-their-way-to ..., babies are conceived, at least for the second time, as needful and as requiring some process of development. If the adult is understood as 'developed,' the baby is understood as 'developing.'

Conceived as potential and thus as proceeding through some process of development, the baby is also understood as naturally possessing whatever it needs to develop, thereby fulfilling its potential. It is within this conception that the notion of 'normal development' finds its home. This is where adult life originates; infancy is the origin of adulthood. For rehabilitation, the original (the infant) is conceived as possessing all that is needed in order to develop its full potential of adulthood.

From this spring the conceptions of the 'good birth' and the 'healthy newborn.'[3] Counting the fingers, counting the toes, etc., of a newborn represents our concern and desire for a 'healthy baby,' which, in turn, represents our desire to produce an infant who is capable of developing normally into an adult. One requirement for this development is that the infant possess the potential for sense perception. Normal development requires that the infant have all of its five senses and have them in good working order. It is in this way that infants are conceived as the origin of adulthood.

We can now understand how the presence of blindness, a sense in non-working order, becomes interesting for rehabilitation. Blindness means that it *cannot* develop normally, and thus its particular potential for adulthood is at risk. The blind baby is interpreted as missing one of the necessary conditions for such development. The interest now is to minimize the risk for the fulfilment of potential and to compensate, in one way or another, for the lack of the sense of sight.

There is, however, something else that contributes to rehabilitation's interest in blind infants and blind children. As potential adults, infants are understood by rehabilitation in terms of 'promise.' They hold the promise of adulthood. (This view is held by adulthood in general.) Rehabilitation's 'real' interest is adulthood insofar as it is committed to providing assistance, wherever it might be needed, to infants and children in fulfilling their potential and promise. Infants and children are promising inasmuch as they represent the promise for the continuation and reproduction of adulthood. They represent the promise of the continuation of a family name; they represent the promise of 'great works' in the arts, sciences, and humanities; they represent, too, the promise of righting the wrongs of current and past generations; they represent discovery, seeing what has heretofore remained unseen, producing what has not yet been produced, creating new and better ways to replace the old, and the like. Children represent the promise for a human condition that surpasses and is better than current and past ones. This is why, like any adult, rehabilitation is interested in children and why it takes care of them.

We can see now that rehabilitation is committed to *itself* insofar as it understands infants and children as holding the promise for adulthood. We see also that rehabilitation is committed to establishing the proper conditions for the potential fulfilment of this promise. One of these proper conditions is the proper working condition of the senses. Whatever other conditions are required for adulthood, the rehabilitation of

3 I address this issue specifically in 'The Birth of Disability' (Michalko 1987).

blind children and infants presupposes the sense of sight as a necessary condition. But if rehabilitation understood sight as necessary, why would it be committed to working with blind infants? Since it does, rehabilitation must have some way to deal with this missing necessary condition.ˆ

Fraiberg develops 'sighted-child ranges.' These ranges are necessary for comparison. There is a *need* to compare the development of sighted children with that of blind children. This comparison suggests that rehabilitation holds the view that blind children *potentially* hold the same promise for adulthood that sighted children do. The promise that blind children have is the promise that they *can* be as promising as the promise held in sighted children. Rehabilitation holds that blindness *can* be as promising as sightedness. Fraiberg's educational program must develop practices and procedures that will result in blind children acquiring 'advantage,' where such advantage means that their development is comparable to that of sighted children.

The notion of comparison is crucial. For Fraiberg, the development of a blind child can never be the *same* as that of a sighted child. It can only be comparable. Her educational program allows for a developmental range for blind children that comes 'close' to the developmental range of sighted children. Even if a blind child has the advantage of Fraiberg's program, she or he will acquire an advantage not *equal* to that of a sighted child but one that is only comparable, that only comes *close*. Thus rehabilitation also promises something. It promises that any blind child who avails him- or herself of the practices of rehabilitation will come *close* to being as promising as a sighted child. But what is most interesting is that rehabilitation claims that its practices allow a blind child to come as close to seeing as possible. Rehabilitation promises blindness a closeness to sight. It promises blindness an 'intimacy' with sight.

Rehabilitation's version of intimacy comes in the form of the 'shadow.' Its version of intimacy is steeped in a particular version of the relation between the original and its image. We have already spoken about how rehabilitation conceives blindness as a shadow of sight and how it conceives sight as the original. Sight is understood as the way things 'should be' and how they should be this way 'from the beginning.'

But there is still another way in which sight is conceived as original. In common-sense and scientific terms – it is interesting to note that, in this respect, both hold the same view – sight is conceived as that sense which provides for much of what we know about the world. Knowing the world hinges to a great extent upon seeing it. I have already shown in chapter 2 how our everyday language is infused with visual metaphor as a way to reference not only ability but also knowledge. The adage 'Seeing is believing' means just that; sighted persons *truly* believe what they see. There is a certainty that comes along with seeing. Conversely, our everyday language is infused with the metaphor of blindness as a way to make reference to inability, lack of knowledge, and uncertainty.

The discipline of rehabilitation knows this about seeing and not seeing and knows it only too well. This is what rehabilitation programs focus on. They evoke the notion, for example, of 'concept development.' This refers to how seeing infants and children tacitly become familiar or intimate with their environment. They learn that ceilings meet walls, the size, shape, and colour of objects; they learn, too, that persons can be distinguished from one another based on their physical features, and the rest. Learning such things leads to knowing the world in a taken-for-granted way. This is the 'natural way' of things.

Blind children are another story. Their blindness prevents them from learning these things in a tacit way and thus prevents them from ever taking the world for granted. Rehabilitation claims that blind children must *explicitly* learn these things if there is any hope for them to learn about their world and any hope for them to fulfil their promise.

Thus blindness raises the 'problem of knowledge.' There is certainly some connection between seeing and knowing. The fact that persons who see take their sight and subsequent knowledge for granted attests to this connection. Blind persons, too, evoke this connection in the living of their lives.

To the extent that the expression 'sighted world' makes reference to this connection, the world *is* indeed sighted. Seeing and sight provide, in part, for the experience and understanding of a world-in-common. They provide for the possibility of the public realm. This means that seeing and sight contribute to the transcendence of private experience through the invocation of the possibility of the realm of public experience. Blindness does represent, from the point of view of this public realm, not only the possibility but also the threat of entrapment in private experience.[4] Blindness does represent a threat to the dialogue between private and public life – a dialogue mediated by the transcendental character of a world-in-common. Blindness is often a potentially privatizing experience. Such an

---

4 I am greatly indebted to the late Stephen Karatheodoris for this idea. He and I spent several hours in conversation regarding, what we called, the 'problem of blindness.' Stephen and I conducted a year of research together on blindness during the early 1980s. In living my life as well as in writing this book, I always keep in mind his admonition to me: 'Always look for the blind soul.'

understandiñg is socially derivative insofar as it springs from the ways in which blindness is conceived and practised in our society.

The privatization that comes from blindness is not the privacy engendered by solitude, loneliness, or even alienation. It is more radical than this insofar as it is marked by isolation from the outside world and by an imprisonment in *one's own self.* The privacy engendered by blindness is the privacy created by exclusion. It is the privacy created by exclusion from a world-in-common and thus an exclusion from any dialogue between private and public life. It is the privacy faced by those who take their own experience to be the only experience as a result of exclusion from the outside world, from the public realm. The public realm is exclusionary to the extent that it does not *accept* private experience unless it can be transformed into the shareable public experience of a world-known-in-common. The public realm expects, indeed demands, that persons *accept* their private experience as just that, private, and thus necessarily excluded from public experience. This is why it is so often said that blind persons must 'accept their blindness.' This means that blind persons must accept their blindness as a privatizing experience, as a world not shared in common, and an experience *not* to be included in the world.[5]

Let me dramatically illustrate this. I spent some time speaking with a three-year-old blind boy, Mark, at his home. We sat on the floor, legs spread in front of us, rolling a ball back and forth. At one point, the ball hit Mark's foot and bounced away from us. Mark immediately began trying to locate the ball. He began 'looking' for the ball by stretching his arms out very quickly in as many directions as he could.

After a short time, Mark stopped 'looking' and said, 'My mommy could find the ball.' 'Really?' I replied. 'Yeah,' Mark said, ' 'cause she can see.' I asked, 'How do you know that?' Without any hesitation, Mark answered, ' 'Cause she's got really, really, really long arms!'

What do we make of such an exchange, particularly Mark's last utterance? Considering Mark's age, we may certainly find his remark to be

---

5 Blindness is certainly included in the world insofar as its recognition is possible only in the world. Its inclusion, however, is limited to its appearance and to making its appearance topical. But as a legitimate, favoured, preferred, or choice-worthy experience, blindness is not included. This is why blind persons must continuously *deny* their 'visual experience' and conceive of it as defective and, why they must deny their experience as a way to recognize the 'right' experience of sight. 'Imagining the point of view of the other,' therefore, is strictly a one-way imagination. Blind persons *must* imagine the point of view of sighted others, but sighted persons *cannot* imagine a blind point of view.

cute. Any child's behaviour is regarded as cute when it is interpreted as an attempt to imitate adult behaviour. It is especially cute when it is interpreted as an attempt to explain complicated human affairs. But, when we consider Mark's blindness, we find a certain sense of pathos in his remark. We see Mark, not only as exhibiting the cuteness of a child, but also as a blind child. We are tempted to enjoy the cuteness of Mark's explanation regarding what it is to see, and yet our joy is tempered with a sense of pathos. We experience the ambivalence that resonates between joy and pathos when we hear Mark's answer to my question.

Children's cuteness is temporary and there is an expectation that they will grow out of it. Their childlike explanations of the world will mature into adult understandings. But for now, they are cute. However, the maturation of a blind child is not so certain. When we hear Mark's answer, we also hear a 'What if ...?' 'What if' Mark says, and indeed believes, the same thing when he is ten years of age, or eighteen, or twenty-five, or ...? For now, the cuteness of his answer resonates with pathos created by our anguish of this 'What if ...?'

Rehabilitation also hears the cuteness and the pathos in Mark's answer. Its temptation, however, is different from ours. Whereas we are tempted to hear only cuteness, rehabilitation is tempted to hear only pathos. In Mark's answer, rehabilitation hears the privatizing nature of blindness created by an exclusion from the world known through sight. The sighted child will learn what it means to see as he or she grows older and will then take this for granted. But the blind child ... How will she or he learn what it means to see? What if Mark continues to believe that seeing means the ability inherent in really long arms? Despite the fact that sight cannot see itself, how will Mark come to know, without sight, that seeing and arms are not the same? How will Mark come to know the outside world, the outside 'sighted' world – the world from which he is excluded by virtue of his blindness? How will he come to know that his private experience of seeing as really long arms is not a common experience and does not belong in the public realm? How will Mark come to know that the world is seen and seeable? How will he function in this world – this world that excludes him in the most pervasive way possible? How can he avoid the pathetic life of exclusion?

It is questions such as these that drive rehabilitation to hearing only pathos in Mark's answer. The single most overriding concern of rehabilitation is to programmatically intervene in Mark's life in a way that will result in Mark's achieving a closeness and an intimacy with sight. The intention of rehabilitation is to give blind children the opportunity to understand their privatizing experience as illusion. Thus the only hope for a blind child resides in 'getting to know' sight, coming close to it and becoming intimate with it. Blindness can escape its imprisonment in itself by including itself in the 'world of sight' through developing a closeness and intimacy with it. Blindness can now shadow sight and cling to it in a way that only the love which comes from intimacy can.

But there is something perverse about this intimacy and the love it engenders. This intimacy is developed through 'getting to know' the outside world by making it an object of inquiry. Mark and other blind children, with the help of rehabilitation, turn sightedness and the sighted world into an object of study and, through this study, get to know it. Unlike seeing children, who develop an intimacy with sight by 'living it,' blind children develop this intimacy by studying it. Seeing children come to love seeing through the intimacy of sensual experience. Blind children come to love seeing through the intimacy that comes from studying an object. Seeing children come to love their seeing and sightedness through the sensual finality of experience, whereas blind children come to love sightedness only through the adolescent version of love, which is infatuation. Blindness is infatuated with sight. Like anyone who is infatuated, blindness can only cling. Sightedness moves through the world with a sensual finality, experiencing itself as an essential part of that world. Blindness, on the other hand, moves through the world clinging to it with an objective finality, *accepting* itself as essentially excluded from that world.

The cuteness and the pathos that Mark's response elicits notwithstanding, it represents a depiction of touch as the distance sense.[6] Hearing and smell also play a role in experiencing distant objects, but it is the sense of touch which brings those objects into the immediate experience of contact. Mark may have heard the ball bounce off his foot, and he certainly felt it. Hearing did play a role in Mark's experience of the ball as 'somewhere in the distance.' But contact with the distant object (the ball) was, for Mark, *dependent* upon the sense of touch. Eyesight was irrelevant to him. Touch was the most crucial distance sense for Mark. What he needed for contact with the ball was longer arms and not eyesight.

Diderot (1982, 77–8) speaks of this need in his 'Letter on the Blind for the Use of Those Who See':

---

6 There has been an interesting development together with a growing body of literature in the area of the senses defined under the rubric of the 'anthropology of the senses.' See, for example, Howes 1991, Synnott 1993, Leder 1990, and Classen 1993. Howes provides an excellent introduction to this work, along with a collection of many of its exemplars.

One of our company bethought him of asking our blind man if he would like to have eyes. 'If it were not for curiosity,' he replied, 'I would just as soon have long arms: It seems to me my hands would tell me more of what goes on in the moon than your eyes or your telescopes; and besides, eyes cease to see sooner than hands to touch. I would be as well off if I perfected the organ I possess, as if I obtained the organ which I am deprived of.'

Eyesight is a curious thing for persons who are blind, especially for those who are congenitally blind. In fact, blind persons are more curious about eyesight than are those who see. Persons who see typically take eyesight for granted and are not curious about it or about their seeing. Curiosity occurs only when eyesight cannot be taken for granted, such as when blindness occurs or when someone does not see in the same way she or he did before. But, for the most part, curiosity about eyes is restricted to those who experience the 'mystery of the eye' through the 'shadow of blindness.'

Except for curiosity, Diderot's blind man would rather not have eyes. He would rather have 'long arms.' This blind man imagines what he would be given were he given eyes. Eyes would *give* him the ability to experience distant objects such as the moon. The gift of eyes would endow him with the possibility of adventure that springs from an expanded universe (Levin 1988, 56). The blind man's world, now spatially framed by his body (his reach), his hearing, and his sense of smell, would be expanded were he to have eyes. With eyes, and their enhancement by telescopes, he could even have in his sensual experience an object as distant as the moon. The blind man has a sense of this and thus knows, without seeing, that eyes essentially claim the ability to give him the experience of distance. Even though he is curious about this claim, the blind man rejects the gift of eyes.

He rejects this gift on the basis that his sense of touch can tell him more about distant objects than can eyes. What can eyes tell him about the moon other than that it is there? This, the blind man already knows. Eyes can tell him what the moon 'looks like.' They can tell him what the moon 'appears to be.' That the moon has an appearance, the blind man knows. But eyes cannot tell him what 'goes on in the moon.' To know this would require more than eyes. The blind man knows that appearances do not necessarily reveal what goes on behind them.[7] This requires contact with what appears. The blind man implies that it is necessary to 'come in touch' with an appearance in order to see what lies behind it and to see what makes it appear in the way that it does. This cannot be done with eyes alone. Seeing may be believing, but it is not necessarily knowing. Diderot's blind man is articulating what Berger (1963, 23) calls the 'first wisdom' of sociology, namely, 'things are not what they seem.' Eyes allow *only* the seeing of what 'seems to be' (Arendt 1971, 38).

The second basis upon which the blind man rejects the gift of eyes is that they cease to see before hands cease to touch. Without coming in touch with them, eyes only see appearances, only what seems to be. Appearances, such as the moon when seen only with the eyes, come and go. When appearances disappear, we can keep them only through visual memory (Taussig 1993), and, like appearances themselves, memories fade. Eyes require the assistance of memory; otherwise, they cease to see. The blind man suggests that touching is another matter. Touching brings appearances *to* oneself. The self is now 'in touch' with the appearance. Touching symbolizes inquiry and a coming to know what lies behind appearances and what they rely on for their appearance. Touching can provide a sense of 'what is going on' in appearances. This knowledge is sustained even after appearances are 'out of reach.' But what sustains it, is not memory only. Instead, it is sustained by the desire to 'be in touch' with appearances, with one's world, and by the wisdom that things are not what they seem. *This* continues long after memory fades and eyes cease to see. Curious as he is, Diderot's blind man rejects the gift of eyes in favour of longer arms.

Diderot's blind man suggests that he would be as well off perfecting what he already has than receiving what he does not. He already has hands, arms – a sense of touch. He favours perfecting this over having eyes. What would be more perfect than longer arms? He treats longer arms 'as if'[8] they would give him something of which he is now deprived. Longer arms would 'put him in touch' with more of his world. What he is in touch with is limited by the length of his arms. Longer arms would address this limit. The blind man knows that there is more to be in touch with. He knows that appearances are constantly and continuously appearing and disappearing. Eyes would tell him nothing that he does not

7 Arendt (1971, 19–26) speaks of the invisible in the visible; that is, of what resides in appearances but cannot be seen with the eye. This stems from Plato's cave metaphor (*Republic*, book 7).

8 Arendt (1982, 65) connects the 'as if' to imagination and judgment. This is precisely what Diderot's blind man does. He imagines that longer arms would put him in touch with 'what goes on' in the world and judges this gift as having a far greater value than the 'natural gift of vision.'

already know, and they would not reveal what lies behind appearances, either those he can now touch or those which eyes would permit him to 'see.' The blind man seeks to know what goes on behind appearances. Perfecting his touch is the only thing that will help him in his quest. Eyes would be of no help.

Like Diderot's blind man, Mark wishes he had longer arms. He could then find the ball. Finding it means that Mark is 'in touch with it.' He would have the ball in his grasp and in his world. Eyes would be of no help to him in this quest. They would allow him merely to 'see the ball.' Eyes would not *give* the ball to Mark's world. Even if he had eyes that could see, Mark would have to move to the ball (lengthen his arms) in order to 'be in touch with it.' Mark's mother is able to 'hand him the ball.' The ball passes from her hand to his, from her touch to his. Like Diderot's blind man, Mark treats longer arms 'as if' they would give him something of which he is now deprived.

Conceiving 'seeing' as 'really, really, really long arms' allows Mark to imagine his mother as possessing the ability to be in touch with the ball even though it is out of his reach. This is not the case for Diderot's blind man. For him, the moon is out of reach for everyone, blind or not. Eyes can certainly see the moon. Even so, those who do see the moon with their eyes assume that they are not seeing everything. They assume that there is more to see than what is seen with their eyes. They 'see' that eyes need help to see the moon. Thus, a telescope. But this 'seeing' is not something they see with eyes or even with telescopes.

Diderot's blind man 'sees' this as well. He sees that the telescope enhances the ability of eyes. Enhanced or not, this ability does not bring objects as distant as the moon into reach. The telescope thus does not give eyes the thing of which they are deprived. Diderot's blind man already knows that the moon is there. Eyes might refine his knowledge, and he is curious about this, but they would not give him anything of which he is now deprived; they would not put the moon 'in his reach.' Eyes would not 'guide' him to an understanding of what goes on in the moon.

Let me now illustrate the connection between blindness and imagination. Several years ago, I was conducting research regarding the mainstreaming or, what is often called, the 'integration' of blind elementary school students. As part of this project, I visited a fourth-grade classroom where one of the students was blind. Jonathan was nine years old and had been totally blind since birth. Along with the twenty-three students, there were three adults in the classroom. I was there, of course, and so was the classroom teacher. At that time, the school board engaged itinerant teachers specially educated to teach blind and visually disabled students. These itinerant teachers would travel from school to school and assist classroom teachers in teaching their disabled students. The itinerant teacher was also present.

During the course of my visit, the classroom teacher conducted an exercise with her students that consisted in asking them what they would like to do as adults in terms of a career. It was a more sophisticated version of the question What would you like to be when you grow up? There were several responses. Some of the students wanted to be nurses, others doctors, still others police officers, some fire-fighters, and one student (a boy) wanted to be an astronaut. As for Jonathan, he said he wanted to become a truck driver.

Shortly after this exercise, the students were sent out of the classroom for their recess period. At that point, the itinerant teacher asked Jonathan to stay back in the classroom. When the other children had left, the itinerant teacher explained to Jonathan that he could not become a truck driver since he was blind. Jonathan simply responded, 'I know.' The teacher then called Jonathan's 'buddy' back into the classroom, and Jonathan and his buddy went out for recess. The itinerant teacher then explained to the classroom teacher and me that 'you just can't give these kids false expectations. It's really unrealistic and then they just don't have a realistic sense of the world.' Neither the itinerant teacher nor the classroom teacher suggested that becoming an astronaut was equally unrealistic. When I mentioned it, both teachers laughed, and the itinerant teacher said, 'But at least it's possible.'

The itinerant teacher felt that she was acting responsibly when she reminded Jonathan of the unrealistic character of his vocational aspiration. She did not want Jonathan to develop 'false expectations' – expectations that Jonathan, because of his blindness, could and should not 'realistically' expect. Unwittingly, the teacher was *teaching* Jonathan about sight; she was teaching him that truck driving was an activity reserved, not for him, but for those, like those who want to become astronauts, who can see. But Jonathan seemed to already know this. I suppose Jonathan was evoking his imagination as a way to respond to the exercise and was speaking more about what he *wanted*, rather than what he was *able*, to become. I suppose the other children were responding in the same way. Raising the spectre of false expectation suggests that one faculty whose development is understood as a detriment to blind children is 'imagination.'[9]

This is difficult to understand since it is the faculty of imagination that will allow, especially congenitally blind children, to 'get to know' sight – to imagine what it means to see. We saw that Mark, at three years old, was already beginning to develop a sense of this meaning through imagining sight as 'really, really long arms.' But we also saw how this imaginative relation to the idea of sight is troublesome to rehabilitation. It is this troublesome character of imagining what it means to see that prompts the itinerant teacher to remind Jonathan that he *cannot* become a truck driver. Imagination, too, is conceived here as troublesome unless it is realistic and hence no longer imaginative. Yet, Mark, Jonathan, and other blind children rely heavily upon their imaginations to develop a version of what it means to see. It is this faculty that rehabilitation seeks to discipline through the invocation of control via an overly concretized version of seeing conceived as sheer ability, or better, as 'sheerability.' This rehabilitative practice privileges the public character of seeing through emphasizing the 'de-abilitating' character of the privacy of blindness.

Jonathan was acting, from the point of view of rehabilitation, 'as if' he was experiencing sight rather than knowing sight. Academics often receive a similar reminder to the one Jonathan did. They are often chided for speaking on behalf of an experience they are studying as though they experienced it. I am speaking of those academics involved in the ethnographic method of research, which makes use of various observational techniques but especially that of participant observation. Even in the case of this latter technique, academics are often reminded to speak *only* of their observations and not of their participation insofar as the object of their study is not available or accessible to them by way of participation. Thus academics who ethnographically study cultures, subcultures, social settings, and the like speak only of their observations insofar as they are not full-fledged and *bona fide* members of those settings. To turn Wittgenstein's phrase somewhat, we might say, 'Of that which we do not experience, we cannot speak.'

9 It might be argued that blind persons are more concerned with adjusting to the world than they are with imagination. They must become educated, find jobs, build friendships, and so on, in a world that presents many obstacles to them and even discriminates against them. This argument suggests that imagination should be put on hold until these survival needs are taken care of. But, any need to survive is always animated by an 'imagined world' which inevitably follows survival. Thus imagination is crucial, especially for blind children.

Those academics who do speak about a social setting they are studying as if they experienced it are often described as 'going native.' Although available as a characterization for academics, it is not possible to characterize Jonathan in this way. For Jonathan to be characterized as going native would require him to acquire the ability to see. 'Coming close' to sighted-child ranges, as Fraiberg would have it, is not good enough. Jonathan can come close to sight but cannot become sight. Ethnographers can come close to membership in a social setting but cannot become members. Membership means that a setting and how it works are taken for granted. It is this taken-for-grantedness that ethnographers seek to topicalize and, in their various ways, study. Jonathan, like the ethnographer, is engaged in developing the need to topicalize and study the taken-for-granted character of seeing. Jonathan, like the ethnographer, who spends a lifetime studying a culture, may eventually have more to say about the 'culture of sight' than those who spend a lifetime living this culture. This is dependent upon Jonathan's decision to live reflectively or not as a blind person in the 'country of the sighted.'

Thus experience is the best teacher, but this is so only if we let it teach us. Jonathan may learn much from his experience with seeing and sight but will do so only if he chooses to live imaginatively. Jonathan himself can become a teacher insofar as he could have much to say to those who see about what it means to see. Jonathan could teach insofar as he could choose to live reflectively with his blindness in the midst of seeing and, therefore, learn from the fact that it is *impossible* to live with sight in a taken-for-granted way. We can rephrase Karatheodoris's question What is blindness? and ask, What can blindness teach us?

Rehabilitation, too, asks this question. But the lesson it learns is unimaginative. It learns that the good life is the life of seeing and that it is vulnerable to distortion and to its possible consequence of nightmarish disaster. Rehabilitation learns this and this only – it learns that blindness, as a point of view and as a life, is distorted and limited. It learns that the only view that blindness provides is one of distortion and that the only life blindness can offer is one limited by lack. Rehabilitation seeks to restore the condition of blindness to its original and proper condition as a way to ameliorate these negative conditions. It seeks to teach blindness about sightedness so that it can come to know sightedness and, equally importantly, so that blindness can come to know itself as the distorted shadow of sight. Rehabilitation seeks to teach blindness not only about its limits but also *that* it is limited in relation to the standard of sight.

Recall that Nunez had a similar relation to blindness in 'The Country of the Blind.' Soon after he stumbled into this country, he realized that the physical world of these people was limited by the mountains surrounding their valley. Nunez also realized that the people in the country of the blind were able to master their physical environment through an exaggerated development of their other senses. He quickly came to see that these people had no word in their language for sight nor did they have a concept of it. He was surprised that the citizens were not interested in coming to know sight. Nunez was most astonished in this country because its people believed that what was real to them was real to anyone and was not a distortion.

Because he could see, Nunez knew better. He could see what the blind people could not. Although Nunez admired how the people adjusted to a physical reality they could not see, he knew that they were indeed adjusted to blindness. Soon after his arrival, Nunez began to interpret his presence in this country as an opportunity to teach the citizens about the world that they could not see and hence could not know. But the people were not interested in knowing about his 'sight' and did not believe his claims to knowing reality.

Finally, something happened – something which Nunez knew all along would. Disaster struck. The mountains began to fall. Nunez, however, was able to escape. At the last moment, he climbed out of the quagmire of the country of the blind into the enlightened safety of the country of the sighted. And he managed to take Medina-sarote with him. She followed Nunez, her love, up from the country of the blind, clinging to him for her life with all of her might.

Even though Nunez could not foresee the collapse of the mountain, he knew that disaster was pending. He knew that the privatization that comes with blindness, in this case, the imprisonment of the country of the blind within itself, would ultimately lead to disaster regardless of the form it would take. He also knew that the life of the people in this country was not the public life of the *agora* or of the metropolis. The country of the blind represented the prison that comes from an experience trapped within itself. Nunez was aware that privacy which experiences only itself is doomed. The country of the blind represented the extreme consequence of individual privatization. It represented the t(error) of mistaking private life for all of life. But Nunez could take some solace in knowing that at least one citizen of the country of the blind was infatuated by sight; and that this infatuation allowed her to escape the prison of her privacy, which permitted her an intimacy with sight, an intimacy to which she clung for her life.

Rehabilitation is not so different from Nunez, at least in terms of orienting to disaster. Rehabilitation assumes that if Mark continues to believe that seeing means having really, really long arms and that if Jonathan continues to believe that he can become a truck driver, disaster, in one form or another, will strike. This disaster is twofold. First, there is the disaster that comes with dashed expectations, especially when such expectations are developed falsely in the first place. This is the disaster that comes to anyone whose action is oriented to a belief system which is false. If Jonathan believes that he can become a truck driver, he will experience at least some disappointment when he is shown that his belief is in fact false. Second, there is the disaster that comes to those who find certain experiences to be inaccessible to them, especially when they expect these experiences to be accessible. This is the adolescent version of disaster that comes from being excluded on the basis of being different, that is, on the basis of not being 'like everyone else.' Many adolescents experience the disaster of being rejected from certain groups because of some difference. This is the adolescent version of the value of belonging to a collective, where what is desired is the desired look of the collective. Each adolescent desires to look like every other adolescent.

For blind persons, the most disastrous thing is the inaccessibility of *their* world to those who can see. No one who can see can ever be part of a blind person's experience, or, in Wells's terms, no one who can see can ever become a citizen in the country of the blind. If we take Nunez's position, who would want to? Who would want to live without the sensual experience of the sense of sight? Who would want to participate in the life of a blind person when that life and that person interpreted what they 'saw' as real? Who would want to participate in Mark's life if, at age twenty-five, he believed sight to be really, really long arms? For rehabilitation, for Nunez, and, indeed, for anyone who can see, and I include here, ironically, blind persons as well, blindness is *not* an experience at all; instead, it is the nihilistic missing of the *real* experience, which is the sensual finality of seeing.

This is the disaster that rehabilitation orients to and tries to prevent by restoring the blind person's interpretation of the world to the 'proper' interpretation which comes through seeing. This is why rehabilitation 'trains' blind persons, especially those who are congenitally blind, to interact with others under the rubric of 'sighted interaction.' Blind persons are encouraged to use phrases such as 'I saw,' 'see you later,' 'I saw him yesterday,' and the like.

The most striking example of such practices I experienced was during my observation of a rehabilitation class conducted by a rehabilitation teacher with a nineteen-year-old woman who was totally blind from birth. The overall program was called 'Adjustment to Blindness,' and the particular class was called 'Activities of Daily Living.' The lesson on this day was to teach the young woman, Jennifer, to 'look' toward the voice of the person with whom she was speaking. The rehabilitation teacher, Lynn, explained to Jennifer that this technique would enable her to make 'eye contact,' something she said sighted persons value. Lynn went on to explain that 'people get nervous when they are talking to you and your head is rolling and you're looking all around. You have to make eye contact and show them that you look just like them.'

Lynn's concern was that Jennifer's world would be inaccessible to someone who could see. The lack of eye contact would make sighted persons nervous and, presumably, would put an end to any further 'comfortable' interaction. When Lynn told Jennifer that she had to show sighted persons that she was 'just like them,' Lynn was not speaking literally. The achievement of eye contact would not make Jennifer sighted, and not being sighted means that she is not 'just like them.' Lynn must have meant something else and must have assumed that Jennifer would understand. What Lynn must have meant was that Jennifer has to 'work' at demonstrating that she is not imprisoned in the experience of her blindness. Jennifer can be 'just like them' if she can show that her blindness is not only privatizing: to this end, eye contact while speaking with sighted persons.

But making eye contact turns out to be more difficult than it initially seems. At one point during their session, Lynn said, 'No. Now you're staring.' 'Staring, what do you mean?' was Jennifer's reply. Lynn explained, 'Well, you have to look away once in a while. Otherwise you're staring and that makes people nervous.' After a brief discussion, Lynn suggested to Jennifer that she should 'probably look away about every five seconds.' Lynn then added, 'But don't make it five seconds every time because that would look too automatic.'

Thus the simple act of eye contact during conversation turns out to be not so simple, whether we are blind or not. The interactional accomplishment of 'eye contact' raises notions such as staring, glancing, nervousness, and the rest. Jennifer's lesson raised the idea of what eyes do other than see and what could be done with eyes other than look. This lesson began to teach Jennifer another side to eyes. There are stares and cold stares, glances and penetrating glances, eyes that reveal and eyes that tell nothing, looks that are friendly and warm and looks that kill, and all of these emanate from the side of eyes that goes beyond the realm of physio-logical function into the realm of the mysterious. Jennifer did learn tech-niques for engaging in conversations with sighted persons, but her lesson provided the occasion for her to learn much more. The opportunity was there for Jennifer to 'glimpse' the mystery of the eye wrapped as it is in its sensual signification.[10] Alas, mystery was not part of Jennifer's lesson. The demystification of the mystery of human interaction through the invoca-tion of technique was the only lesson of the day. The seeds of mystery were planted, intentionally or not, and Jennifer now has the possibility of cultivating this mystery on each and every occasion of interaction with sightedness.

I am not suggesting that Jennifer actually learned the lesson of the 'mystery of the eye'; nor am I suggesting that Jennifer did not need to learn various techniques involved in the 'activities of daily living.' What I am suggesting is that these latter techniques are necessary but that buried in the techniques themselves is the deeper lesson of mystery. Techniques are not in and of themselves complete or sufficient. If we dig through the surface of any technique, we will find the values, principles, and standards that orient these techniques and make them possible in the first place. We already saw, in Jennifer's lesson, that eye contact could not be totally captured solely by technique. An attempt to do so is what led Lynn and Jennifer to the problem of staring and nervousness. Try as they might to find one, there did not seem to be an obvious technical solution to this problem.

Any rehabilitation project which relies solely on technique remains incomplete and insufficient, thus leading to its own form of disaster, namely, eyes without mystery. Rehabilitation must provide technique to blind persons, but it must provide more. Rehabilitation needs to learn the lesson that it must create a need in its clients that it cannot satisfy. It must create the need in blind persons to raise the problem of the essen-tial incompleteness of seeing and thus retain the mystery of the eye. This is a problem to which there is no solution, but it must be continually raised. Rather than seeking a technical solution to this non-technical problem, rehabilitation, together with blind persons, must raise the prob-

10 I read Bataille (1985, 17) as alluding to what I have called the 'mystery of the eye.' He says, 'It seems impossible, in fact, to judge the eye using any word other than *seductive*, since nothing is more attractive in the bodies of animals and men. But extreme seduc-tiveness is probably at the boundary of horror.' Mystery is what permits seduction to seduce and horror to horrify. And, there is nothing more mysterious than the cohabita-tion of the two in one look.

lem of the mystery of the eye as something which provides for the possibility of a thoughtful life. Once the problem of the mystery of the eye is artificially solved through technique, there is nothing more for a blind person to do than to search out more and better techniques for living a life. What a blind person ends up with is what Nunez wanted for the people in the country of the blind, namely, to realize that adjusting to a visually inaccessible reality was the only life possible and to realize that excellence in living is to be achieved only in adjusting well.[11] This is precisely why a rehabilitative 'look' at blindness judges the life of a blind person in terms of how intimate he or she is with sight and how well he or she knows sight. Thus rehabilitation's need for 'sighted-child ranges.' The development of a blind child is seen by rehabilitation as the development, in that child, of knowledge regarding sight and techniques for interactionally displaying it. The successful blind person is understood as the one who comes to know that the only reality is the one experienced through sight and is the one who acts 'as if' she or he knows this reality intimately.

Therefore, rehabilitation should develop an ironic relation to the restoration of the condition of blindness. One way to do this is to learn from blindness. It is to allow blindness to teach. Blindness is a disruption to the taken-for-granted ideas and practices of seeing. It does disrupt sight's intimate and familiar, almost familial, relation to the world. Eye contact is not something that is ever explicitly taught to those who can see. They tacitly acquire the ability to make eye contact through the ability to see. Ironically, the ability to make eye contact is derived through making eye contact. This is the lesson that reveals the ironic character of the social world, which rehabilitation and even sightedness can learn from blindness. What rehabilitation can learn from blindness is that sight is a condition cloaked in irony and mystery and thus not achievable solely through the evocation of *techné*. With blindness as its teacher, rehabilitation can learn that *techné* is only part of the picture of sightedness and not the whole of it.

But as Jenny discovered (see chapter 2), rehabilitation sees itself only as teacher and not as student. There is always much, much work to be done. Rehabilitation understands blindness as generating only distortion

---

11 Sacks (1995) relies totally on the notion of 'adjustment' in his discussion of disability. He marvels at the power of adjustment found in the human physiology and, in this, finds nothing to admire or see with wonder except the admirable and wonderful feature of adjustment in the human being.

and error as well as the possibility of the privatizing of experience and subsequent exclusion. There is certainly nothing to learn from this. But there is much to be taught. Teaching, for rehabilitation, takes the form of training and the imparting of techniques. Rehabilitation understands sight as embodied in an 'ideal actor.' This ideal actor is someone who is like every other sighted person insofar as he or she can see, and potentially do, what everyone else can see and do. This ideal actor is an actor who 'fits in' and, ideally, cannot be distinguished from any other actor on the basis of 'looking like' he or she can see. Rehabilitation's ideal actor moves through the world looking like everyone else who sees.

The need for 'fitting in' is what generates rehabilitation's need for the development of 'sighted-child ranges.' These ranges do not make reference to a particular sighted child, but rather to every sighted child. Like any set of ranges, they aim at eliminating any extremes, thereby settling on the middle or the average. These ranges are developed under the auspices of what any sighted child knows and does and not under the auspices of any particular child. They aim at some understanding of 'normal development.'

This is the crux of the matter for rehabilitation. Its animating question is How can our practices be developed such that blind persons can come as close to being normal as possible? The interest here is not in thinking where blindness fits in; instead, the interest is in thinking about how blindness can be *made* to fit in. Rehabilitation's question becomes What does blindness need in order to fit in? This is the question of the adolescent.

If rehabilitation were to achieve a sense of excellence, it would be necessary for it to develop its adolescent interest in the average or in 'looking the same' into the more mature interest of the place of blindness in the world. It would have to think about where blindness fits. It would have to borrow from the ancient Greek idea of *paideia* and 'turn around' the essential nature of blindness. If the essential nature of blindness can be conceived as privatizing experience, rehabilitation would have to turn that nature around, thus demonstrating the possibility of blindness finding and cultivating its place in the world. Rehabilitation would be interested in restoring to blindness the essential need for participation in public life, which blindness often turns around in the face of the privileging of privatizing experience. Blind persons would have to be shown *their* possibility for public life. This involves more than *technē.*

The acquisition of techniques for achieving the 'activities of daily living' offers blind persons only the possibility of 'fitting in' and of coming close to being like anyone else. This leads to a life that continuously monitors itself in relation to how close it can come to doing the things that everyone else does. A life such as this finds the idea of exceptionality repugnant. From this point of view, there is nothing exceptional about a blind person crossing a busy street, nothing unusual about a blind person preparing a five-course meal, or nothing noteworthy about a blind person skiing. There is nothing exceptional about these things since anyone, including blind persons, should do them. It is this orientation that leads to the understanding that persons 'happen' to be blind. Personhood is now essential, while the rest, including blindness, is sheer happenstance.

It is no wonder that blind persons, and rehabilitation as well, often adopt the attitude that it is necessary for blind persons to do as many things as possible, especially when they are conceived of as things done by anyone. This attitude interprets the 'doing of these things' as symbolically representing the 'average life.' It is one way of privileging personhood. It suggests that persons are alike by virtue of personhood. We are alike because we have feelings, hopes and fears, and anxieties; and we are alike because we 'do things.' These 'things' are not 'exceptional things' such as scientific discoveries, literary achievements, athletic accomplishments, or the like. Exceptional things are done by exceptional people. The things rehabilitation celebrates are the ordinary things done by ordinary people – things such as walking down the street, preparing a meal, eating a meal, talking to people, having sex, raising children, *ad infinitum*, if not, *ad nauseam*.

The distinction between what is ordinary and what is exceptional is not always clear for, in the case of blindness, many things are exceptional even though they may appear ordinary. Some blind persons engage in the doing of exceptional things under the auspices that 'ordinary people' are able to do them. Whether or not sighted persons *actually* do them is irrelevant since what is important is that they *can* do them. Here are the words of a man (Parisian 1981, 89) totally blind from birth:

I still feel, at times, that I have to fight and fight and fight to prove things to myself and to others. This can lead to what I call overkill. I'll do things that I probably shouldn't try to do. I'll walk places on my own where I'd be smarter to take an arm. Sometimes I'll do things to the extreme. For example, this fall I insulated my house. After six months of riding transit buses searching for the best insulation system, I finally found one. The procedure I chose meant I had to run vertical steel straps every two feet around my house and then attach a foam board insulation. I did that rotten, tedious job myself using a simple step ladder, a concrete drill and a screwdriver. I'm sure I turned over eight hundred screws. I refused the help that people offered partly because I felt that they would think less of me if I couldn't do it.

Why does Parisian have to continually prove things? Why does he think that people would think less of him? Insulating a house is certainly no ordinary thing, whether done by someone who is blind or not. The difference lies in the notion of 'could.' The conventions of our society hold, and do so quite strongly, that blind persons are incapable of doing many things. The same is not true for persons who see. Parisian lives his life in the face of this convention. He must prove both to others and to himself that he is not ruled by this convention, and he feels that if he were so ruled, 'they,' including himself, would think less of him. Thus Parisian transforms all 'doings,' exceptional or not, into ordinary things. Ordinarily, he *could* do *all* things. Parisian is referring to the 'ordinary conditions' of being human, especially the ordinary condition of sight.

Blind persons often employ the doing of these 'ordinary things' as a way to display their competence and personhood. Doing ordinary things implies that they are done by ordinary people, by anyone, including blind persons, and since we, those of us who are blind, do ordinary things, we are ordinary people. It is this interpretive chain that provides for the basis of accessibility rights by the disability community. Since blind persons do the things everyone else does and are thus persons, they need the right of accessibility. Since people read, blind persons have the right to expect reading material in a format accessible to them. Or, since everyone makes use of public facilities such as restaurants, blind persons have the right to expect restaurants to be accessible.

But much of public life is not accessible to blind persons or to persons with other disabilities. There are many reasons for this, reasons steeped largely in barbaric cultural attitudes and conceptions held about disability. It is this sort of exclusion from public life that generates the development of the orientation toward 'ordinary life' as the 'good life.' The lack of ordinary access or, better, the lack of access to the ordinary is what leads many blind persons, as well as rehabilitators, to doing as many ordinary things as possible and to celebrating ordinary life. Disabled persons need to *achieve* their ordinariness, whereas abled-bodied persons *are* ordinary. This is why no non-disabled person has ever taken a course in 'activities of daily living.'

Many blind persons often use the collective conception that they are unable to perform the ordinary things of life as an occasion to humorously reachieve their personhood. During a conversation among five blind persons, one person said, 'I don't know what they were thinking – I was with my girlfriend, but they thought she was my sister. Then the guy said, "I don't suppose you want drinks?"' Another responded, 'Well, blind people don't drink!' Almost in unison, two others said, 'We don't have sex either, do we?' These remarks were followed by loud laughter from the entire group.

In this example, exclusion from ordinary life is playing itself out in ordinary life. It is obvious that the five blind persons interpreted the situation as one of exclusion. The person (who incidentally was a waiter at a restaurant) who thought the blind patron's girlfriend was his sister and that neither of them would want drinks represented the collective conception that blind persons do not do, at least some, ordinary things. Blind persons do not drink, and they do not have sex.

Even though this story remarks on the pathetic character of some of the prevailing attitudes our culture holds toward disabled persons, there is also an adolescent flavour to it. The comments by the waiter were not directed toward the doing of *any* or *all* ordinary things. The blind person and his girlfriend, who was also blind, did arrive at the restaurant, were seated at a table, and, presumably, were about to order a meal. About these ordinary things, the waiter said nothing. He commented only on the relationship of the two blind people and on drinking. From the point of view of the five blind persons, the waiter commented on the ordinary activities of drinking and sex. It is interesting to note that these two activities are not seen as ordinary in the life of adolescents. Adolescents are not legally permitted to drink, and sex among adolescents is always grist for the commentary mill and, as such, is not considered an ordinary adolescent activity, even today. Drinking and sex are typically conceived of as adult activities. Such activities, when engaged in by adolescents, still produce the titillation that comes from toying with a taboo. Drinking and sex are often experienced and spoken of as extra-ordinary things in adolescent culture, things not yet dampened by the ordinary expectations of everyday adult life. Drinking and sex typically evoke for adolescents the titillation that comes from participating in adult activities while not yet being an adult. It is the mocking of cultural convention.

The group of blind persons were engaged, in a way similar to adolescents, in mocking convention. They were mocking the cultural conception that represents blindness and blind persons as unable to participate *fully* in 'ordinary adult life.' But inability was not restricted to the blind couple in the restaurant. It was in the waiter as well. The waiter could not imagine a way to represent or think of blindness that did not include inability. He could not imagine *himself* as a blind person able to fully participate in life. This lack of imagination often animates interaction between blind and sighted persons. This is why a hairstylist recently asked me, in the midst of cutting my hair, whether or not I lived alone. I am almost certain that this question was never posed by any hairstylist to any sighted customer.

It is this unimaginative relation to *full* participation in life that blind persons, like adolescents, often mock. But unlike adolescents, whom adults imagine as possessing the potential for full participation, blind persons must face, and face all of their lives, the possibility of living with an unimaginative relation, on the part of others, to participation in life. Thus, Parisian needs to 'fight and fight and fight.' Adolescents grow into adults, but blind persons do not grow into sighted persons.

Blind persons may often mock waiters, hairstylists, and anyone else who displays an unimaginative relation to blindness. We who are blind may mock anyone who embodies the cultural conception of blindness as the impossibility of full participation in life. In doing so, we implicitly often mock ourselves. Blind persons, too, grow up in a culture in which blindness is typically conceived as a barrier to full participation in life. When persons 'discover' their blindness (see chapter 3), they, more often than not, discover this barrier. Blind persons believe, and I mean this in the cultural sense, that their blindness is a barrier to full participation in life which often acts to exclude them from public life. If blind persons are 'persons first,' then they are so insofar as, like sighted persons, they harbour the belief and the cultural conception that blindness is, in many ways, exclusionary. Thus, we must 'fight and fight and fight.' Insofar as blind persons mock this belief and cultural conception, they mock persons who see as well as themselves.

Doing the things that everyone else does, being average, is the standard not only for this mocking but also for the rehabilitative enterprise. Rehabilitation aims to restore blindness to its proper and original condition through the development of techniques for daily living as well as the development of technology. The fundamental understanding here is that sight allows persons to do things for themselves in the most natural and taken-for-granted ways. Blindness prevents this. One impulse that is often evoked as a solution to this problem, an impulse steeped in sympathy and charity, is to do things *for* blind persons. The rehabilitative impulse, steeped as it is in the notions of independence and the 'average,' opposes any desire to do things *for* blind persons since such a desire does nothing to restore the condition of blindness. From rehabilitation's point of view, sympathy and charity act only to reinforce the conception that blindness is a hopeless condition and that blind persons are helpless.

Rehabilitation aims to show, through techniques and technology,[12] that blindness is not a hopeless condition and that blind persons are not helpless. It takes this aim seriously. It shows this to *anyone* who is ready to see, including blind persons. Rehabilitation is also serious about the 'readiness' to see. An orientation and mobility instructor told me:

You've got to wait about a month after they lose their sight before you go to see them. It takes the average person about this long to come to terms with their blindness. I mean, after this time, they know they're blind and are now ready to get on with things.

A social worker specializing in work with blind infants and children said,

I do most of my work with the parents. The kids are okay, they're fun. But the parents, well, that's another story. Most of them just aren't ready to see their kids just as kids. They want to do everything for them.

Thus blind persons doing things for themselves is not natural. They must be 'ready' to embrace this idea, which requires both time and work. Blind persons need time to 'come to terms' with their blindness, and parents need 'work' to see their kids as 'just kids.' Seeing blind kids as 'just kids' means that blind kids are just like kids and should do the things that kids do. 'Coming to terms' with blindness means that blindness is now a permanent condition of life, and, if life is to be lived, it is to be lived with that condition.

Being just like kids and coming to terms with blindness require time and work; in particular, personal time and rehabilitative work. Rehabilitation understands itself as an enterprise that does what blind people and parents cannot do, namely, the work required to 'make ready' and prepare blind persons to live 'just like anyone else.' This is the work of orientation and mobility, of activities of daily living, of counselling, and the rest. All of these endeavours see *technē* as the solution to the problem of

13 On the 'question of technology,' Heidegger (1977, 6) says, 'Wherever ends are pursued and means are employed, wherever instrumentality reigns, there reigns causality.' In this sense, rehabilitation conceives technology as 'causing' the conception that blindness is not a hopeless condition. Blindness's *only* hope for not being conceived as a hopeless condition is technology. It is to treat blindness as instrumentally as technology is treated.

blindness. Their answer to Karatheodoris's question What is blindness? is Blindness is a technical problem.

The adolescent nature of rehabilitation stems from two notions: first, rehabilitation understands blindness as the lack of techniques required for daily living; and, second, it understands the successful life as the life that looks like any other life. Just as an adolescent sees the solution to the adolescent problem as the right fashion, the right talk, the right walk, and the rest, rehabilitation sees the solution to the problem of blindness as the right technique for doing the right thing in order to be 'just like ...'

But techniques, and even technology, while raising the question of *how* to do things, beg the question of *what* to make, which is the *real* question of *technē*. Now that I, a blind person, possess techniques and technology, what do I make? What sort of life should I make and live? Not only are techniques unable to answer these questions, they are unable even to raise them. This is the fundamental limit of a commitment to techniques as the solution to the problem of life conceived technically.

Unlike most lives, the life of blindness does bring to light the problem of technique and does so dramatically, so dramatically that we are tempted to fix our gaze solely on that problem. The life of blindness *can* illuminate the problem of life with a light different from the one shed by the need for technique. This is part of a conversation I had with a father of a fifteen-year-old partially sighted, yet 'legally blind,' young man:

Oh! He's fine, he's great. He does everything. I help him, but he builds models of all that stuff. He plays soccer, does track and field and he even does karate. The kid's got ribbons and trophies for all that stuff. He's got friends and everything, and everything's OK. There's always ways you can find to do things even when you can't see hardly anything. He's got all that stuff, he can do all that stuff. But, like he says, who can't? But, you know, you know sometimes there are things you just can't do. He's legally blind and sometimes that hits him right in the face. You know what his biggest problem right now is? Driving! He's fifteen, but no learner's permit. All his friends got 'em. But, not him. Pretty soon his friends will get their licence and some of them already have it. He doesn't know what he's going to do. We've got to deal with this somehow.

Driving, for an adolescent, is crucial and not so merely for the technical purpose of transportation. Driving represents a right of passage; that is, the 'right to drive' represents the beginning of *legitimately* doing the things of adulthood. This is why the driving-age is so crucial to many adolescents. It represents a version of transition from adolescence to adulthood. And it represents more. Driving now becomes one more way of expressing the self. It expresses competence, independence, responsibility, freedom, and many of the other trappings of adult life. Perhaps most importantly, and in the vernacular of the day, driving is 'cool' and so is the driver. Driving speaks volumes in the same mysterious way that the eyes do.

But this adolescent is legally blind and *cannot* drive. There are no techniques available to him which will *enable* him to do so. Only sight will allow him to drive. Even rehabilitation takes a 'back seat' when it comes to the problem of driving for blind persons. Like ophthalmology, rehabilitation too says, 'Nothing can be done.'

The young man must come face-to-face with his blindness. Ironically, rehabilitation must do the same. Driving represents an occasion that compels blind persons to 'look' at their blindness and thus, for the 'first' time once again, compels them to develop a relation to it which raises the problem of answering Karatheodoris's question What is blindness? *This is no technical matter.* Neither technique nor technology can be evoked as a method for developing a relation to blindness since both are *consequences* of such a relation. They are results of particular ways we come to conceive blindness, come to think of it, understand it, and, finally, live it.

As technically competent as he is, this young man will have to face the problem of driving and face it stripped of any technique or technology. Ironically, this was the case all along. *No amount of technique or technology ever made it possible for this young man to think about his blindness.* With the exception of developing more and better techniques, a technical solution to the problem of blindness is final. As final as it is, it does not finalize thinking about blindness.

The need to develop a relation to blindness is a lifelong endeavour, and the only thing that is 'made' is the making and remaking of the problem of blindness. Like life itself, the life of blindness is lifelong. A commitment to technique shortens the life of blindness insofar as it raises and simultaneously solves the problem. Technique is a part of life, but it is not the whole of life. As a part of life, it is natural and even sufficient for technique to both raise and immediately solve the technical part of life. But when blind persons or rehabilitation conceive blindness as *wholly* a technical problem, they are confusing the part for the whole and thus are putting the problem of the life of blindness to rest once and for all. They are acting like Kierkegaard's man who, when asked to entertain himself for the day, finishes at noon. Of those who choose this technical relation to life, Kierkegaard suggests that they are through with life before life is through with them. This is also the case for those of us who are blind. Choosing a technical solution to the problem of blindness means, for those of us who are asked (forced?) to live the life of blindness, that we are through with it before it is through with us.

The adolescent relation to blindness that rehabilitation embodies serves to remind us of our need to develop both a desire and a need to relate to blindness. Answering the question What is blindness? presupposes a preferred and favoured relation to blindness. Buried in our answer is always-already some version of a relation to what blindness means. The quintessential responsibility for both blind persons and rehabilitation is to face blindness *in the face of what they have already made of it.* This is already the beginning of the development of a 'mature' relation to blindness.

I want to look more closely at the idea of adolescence. Adolescence marks the beginning of the recognition of convention. It begins to understand that certain 'natural features,' such as gender, are not so natural. What once seemed natural now seems conventional. The natural, and thus unambiguous, character of male and female now appears conventional and ambiguous insofar as they could at one time be this and at another that. Adolescence marks the beginning of the recognition of the freedom of choice over and against the tyranny of nature. As a way to develop this idea, I turn in the next chapter to a more detailed discussion of the adolescent relation to blindness. I will make use of my own experience of blindness during adolescence as a way to reflect upon this relation. Such a discussion will allow us to *hear* more directly the story of adolescent blindness before listening to what adult blindness has to say.

5

The Gap of Adolescence

When I use the term 'adolescent,' I am not necessarily referring to any specific range of chronological age. This also holds true for my use of any other metaphor which aims at describing or theorizing some idea of the 'life-cycle.' In contrast to chronological usage, I treat these terms as metaphors as a way to think about the various ways we choose to relate to blindness. I do not treat the meaning of blindness as self-evident or unambiguous. Blindness is a choice.

I do not mean that, like Oedipus, we blind ourselves. I am referring to the 'social fact' (Durkheim 1938, 3) that we approach blindness with a conception of it already in hand and that we modify, enhance, and develop this conception through our interaction with it. These choices are at times explicit and at other times implicit, rendering the phenomenon of blindness always, and forever, ambiguous. It is only when we choose to relate to blindness and thus conceive of it in a particular way, that its ambiguity becomes covered over and forgotten in favour of the more certain conception of blindness as clear and self-evident.

I want now to more closely examine the adolescent relation to blindness since it is very tempting to adopt such a relation. Such a relation is seductive insofar as blind persons, their family and friends, as well as the professions of ophthalmology and rehabilitation are often *seduced* into adopting such a relation. Adolescence is interested in appearances, especially when such an interest permits the appearance of any one adolescent to blend into that of any other. Following Baudrillard (1987, 47), we can disappear in appearances and hence reap the promissory harvest of adolescence, which is to be seen without being noticed. We often want our blindness to go unnoticed.

In its life-cycle sense, adolescence is a time when we often want our differences to go unnoticed. Adolescents often want their blindness to disappear and often want to blend into the ubiquity of the appearances of sightedness. This is why blind persons sometimes act 'as if' they can see – an activity sociologists call 'passing.'[1] Blind persons will sometimes pass as sighted persons. With the average as its standard, the adolescent relation to blindness is keenly interested in passing. Its interest is in looking like everyone else and not standing out. Passing is one method for achieving this.

I will examine the phenomenon of passing as it relates to blindness and sightedness, and I will examine it from the point of view of adolescence. I will make use of my own experience of blindness during my adolescence. During this time, my particular story of blindness was a story narrated by the figure of passing. I had less than 10 per cent of so-called normal vision and was referred to, largely by ophthalmologists, in such various ways as 'partially sighted,' 'visually impaired,' 'visually disabled,' and 'visually challenged.' Parenthetically, the historical development of the use of these terms represents the historically shifting conceptions of blindness. Whatever the label, my vision was severely limited and fell within the 'legal' boundaries of blindness. It is this experience that I make use of in this chapter. Along with examining the need to develop an adolescent relation to blindness, I will also introduce the idea of the 'mature passer' as a way to introduce the next chapter. Thus it may seem logical to speak of 'immature' blindness rather than adolescent blindness. Such a term, however, would turn relations to blindness into ontologies. Adolescence captures the flavour of the 'average' and 'looking like everyone else' better than does immaturity. It also permits for the reality of blind persons moving back and forth from one relation to another instead of progressing from one ontology to another.

Let me begin with the work of Goffman. Goffman makes use of what he calls 'impression management' to both raise and understand the sociological problem of passing. He considers the phenomena that make up our social world not as 'natural facts' but instead as 'impressions' which we tacitly manage. Others 'know' that we see if, and *only* if, we create that impression. For those who see, this sort of impression creation and management is not something engaged in consciously but is instead something engaged in tacitly and is never thought about *unless* someone *gets* the impression that someone does not see. Blind persons often make explicit

---

1 I borrow extensively in this analysis from the work of Goffman (1963, 73–90) and Garfinkel (1967, 116–85).

use of these interactional practices of impression management to give the impression that they see or, at least, that they know the world is sighted and know how to act in such a world. In order to pass as sighted, blind persons make use of the taken-for-granted practices of sighted persons.

Goffman (1963, 88) gives the following example of a partially sighted (legally blind) person:

I managed to keep Mary from knowing my eyes were bad through two dozen sodas and three movies. I used every trick I had ever learned. I paid special attention to the colour of her dress each morning, and then I would keep my eyes and ears and my sixth sense alert for anyone that might be Mary. I didn't take any chances. If I wasn't sure, I would greet whoever it was with familiarity. They probably thought I was nuts, but I didn't care. I always held her hand on the way to and from the movies at night and she led me, without knowing it, so I didn't have to feel for curbs and steps.

Even from this brief description, we can get a sense of how attentive the passer must be to even the most ordinary social situations. Persons who see certainly do not pay such close attention to these sorts of situations, if they attend to them at all. Through calculative and attentive interaction, we can produce states of naturalness such as seeing even though that naturalness is not something that comes naturally to us. Whereas blind persons sometimes act as if they can see, sighted persons never intentionally do so since seeing, as well as managing its creation and impression, is something that comes naturally to them.

The person who passes is always aware of social situations and how they are interactionally produced and is thus always aware of what interaction is necessary to fit naturally into them. The passer is naturally attentive and calculative. The need for calculation and attentiveness is generated by the desire to 'fit in,' and, in turn, this desire is generated by the understanding that fitting in is difficult, unexpected, discouraged, or otherwise jeopardized. The desire to fit in is only felt by those who do not feel that they do fit in. This is why passing is such an ubiquitous feature of adolescence.

As a 'legally blind' person, I found adolescence to be a particularly difficult time. This was so since, for much of my adolescent life, I had an overriding concern for normalcy. I wanted desperately to be a normal adolescent and wanted equally as desperately to show others that I was. During this time, I thought of my eye condition as nothing other than abnormal. I knew that I did not fit in, and I knew, too, that if others became aware of my eye condition, they would have thought the same.

Therefore, I led the life of a fully sighted person. I chose to pass. I became a keen observer of social life, attentive to social situations, and readily grasped the calculative feature of social and collective life. My deepest desire was to be, as we said back then, 'one of the guys.'

I grew up in an inner city neighbourhood where 'maleness' was an important and emphasized feature of adolescent life. Driving a car at age sixteen was an expectation that bordered on being compulsory, especially for 'boys.' This expectation was not quite as rigid for 'girls.' The ability and right to drive a car at age sixteen were a normal expectation in my neighbourhood. Everyone in my neighbourhood expected sixteen-year-old boys to drive. This presented me with difficulties. It was an extremely tricky situation for me. The desire to drive did not present me with difficulties. I had that and thus did not have to act as if I did. But I had neither the ability nor the right to drive. This is what was tricky, and this is what presented me with difficulties and more insofar as the combination of desiring to drive together with the inability to do so caused me severe personal anxiety.

I did not want to share the fact that I could not drive with my friends since to do so would have amounted to sharing with them the most exclusionary and awful thing about me, namely, that I was abnormal. All along I had acted as if I could see, and admitting that I could not drive because of my eye condition would have amounted to admitting that I was not what I appeared to be, that I was not 'one of the guys.' None of this, however, changed the fact that I could not drive. Somehow this had to be explained. Moreover, the explanation had to maintain my identity as someone who could see. I turned to the social context of my neighbourhood. I used the values, beliefs, conceptions – culture – of my inner city neighbourhood as building blocks for the construction of an explanation that would explain why I was not driving, while at the same time preserving my identity as one of the guys.

As is the case both then and now, many inner city neighbourhoods experience delinquent and quasi-delinquent activity from their adolescent members. This was no different in my neighbourhood. Many of us were engaged in quasi-delinquent activity such as drinking, fighting, and the like. In fact, my neighbourhood *expected* such activity from its 'teenagers.' I do not mean that my neighbourhood expected this in a moral sense. It expected such activity insofar as it understood these activities as part of a stage that some adolescents 'went through,' and the expectation was that they would eventually 'grow up' and thus not engage in such activity forever. Anyone who continued such activity into adulthood was understood as someone who did not grow up, as someone who was a criminal or, in the vernacular of my neighbourhood, as someone who was a 'bad actor.' The point is that, in my neighbourhood, adolescent boys saw themselves as 'tough,' and others saw them in the same way. This sort of quasi-delinquent activity was not only expected and acceptable in the ways I have mentioned, but was also understood as appropriate.

It was this social context that I used as the material and building blocks for inventing and constructing a reason, a reason other than blindness, for not being able to drive. My reason for not driving had to fit my inter-actional achievement of a normal adolescent. It had to be a reason that *any* sixteen-year-old boy *could have* for not driving. It had to spring from my identity as a seeing person and not from my identity as a legally blind one. This was my invention, my reason: I invented a story that I was picked up by the police for driving under age and while under the influ-ence of alcohol. This story went on to say that because of this legal charge against me I was not legally allowed to take my driver's test for a year, until I was seventeen years old. This gave me a year's grace, and I would not have to invent another reason for at least one year.

But the invention of this reason through the telling of such a story is not as simple as it might seem. My story could not be told in any effective way through one telling. I needed my friends and acquaintances to orient to me not only as a person who did not drive but as one who did not drive for a 'good reason.' Like any good reason, my reason for not driving had to come from a legitimate source and thus not come from me alone. I needed my story to be told not only by me but by others. I told my story to only two or three of my closest friends. I then relied on the 'grapevine' which existed in my neighbourhood for the rest. Soon, my story was being told by everyone.

Getting others to tell your story is not as simple as it might seem. The elaborate grapevine aside, I had to provide the opportunity for others to tell my story. At parties, I would often initiate discussion about driving, especially with those who did not know that I did not drive. 'Driving talk' was not unusual in my neighbourhood. During such talk, talk I had initi-ated, my reason for not driving would often naturally evolve. Now, still other people knew.

House parties were almost a ritual in my neighbourhood, and we typi-cally held them on special events such as birthdays, Christmas, New Year's, and the like. Such parties required a certain amount of prepara-tion. We always held them at the house of someone whose parents would be out of town or otherwise engaged. Since we were teenagers, a number of days of preparation were required to arrange for the illegal purchase of alcohol. These preparations complete, we were ready to party.

Most arrived at the party in cars. This did not present any particular difficulty for me since the people in my circle of friends knew that I could not drive and knew why. I always arranged for one of my friends to drive me and my date to the party. For the most part, the strategy worked well. But often my date did not know I could not drive, and the strategy was ineffective. The difficulty this presented was still minimal since 'double dating' was a custom of the times. My inability to drive did not necessarily have to become an issue.

But, I eventually confronted difficulty. This occurred most frequently when the same person accompanied me to several parties. Eventually, as the custom held, it would be my turn to drive. 'Steady dating' meant that my date would have to come to hear my story of why I did not drive. The solution to such a difficulty seems quite simple. I could have just told her. But I could not afford any suspicion being cast my way. Simply volunteering such information would certainly raise suspicion. A direct telling of my story would not do. I had to find the proper situation for such a telling, or, better, I arranged for the situation itself to do the telling. One way to do this, a way I often made use of, was to get someone else to tell my date I could not drive. During the party, and in the presence of my date, I would ask one of my friends to loan me his car. But not just any friend would do. He would have to be a popular person with a reputation for letting others use his car. He would have to be a friend who knew my drunk-driving story. He would also have to be someone who everyone knew wanted to minimize any confrontation with police. He would have to be a friend who would not loan me his car, despite my asking, and a friend who, in the course of my asking, would tell others why he would not loan his car.

This was a tricky way to get the job done. If my friend refused to loan me his car without saying why, I would have to persist until he gave the reason. The danger in this was, of course, that he might break down and loan me the car. But, it was not his car I wanted. This meant that I would have to continually monitor my request until my friend refused by retelling my story. It was this retelling that I was after. I needed to be continuously and constantly in control of the conversation for this to occur. I had to control my own talk as well as that of my friend in order to be seen as a normal, seeing adolescent.

So far I have shown the sort of 'interactional work' that I had to do in order to achieve and maintain some sense of myself as normal and thus ordinary. We can begin to understand the complicated character of such work and to understand, too, the sort of anxiety that accompanies such work. Such anxiety is directly related to the value I had placed on being ordinary. Even though I did not share the normal feature of sightedness with my peers, I did share the value of ordinariness. Like my peers, I desired, almost more than anything else, to be ordinary.

A desire for ordinariness presupposes a particular relation between the self and the other. This means that I had to see my peers as always-already *being* ordinary. From my point of view, if they could see, they were ordinary. I took into account notions such as cliques, who was 'in,' who was 'out,' and the rest. For my purposes then and even now, to a certain extent, all of this *presupposed* sight and *relied* upon it for the possibility of being either 'in' or 'out.' Before I could concern myself with being in or out, I needed to concern myself with its primary requirement – sight.

The 'other' was embodied in individual friends and acquaintances as well as in individual adolescents. But this was only an embodiment, for in a much deeper sense my other was the idea of sight. This was the other I continuously oriented to as the 'good' and do so, at least to some extent, even today. This means that during my adolescence I kept a 'close eye on sight.' I kept a close eye on my peers. I did so in order to come to know the sorts of things I had to do and say so as to achieve sight as the fundamental requirement of ordinariness. But, I kept an eye on them for still another reason. *I needed to know whether or not my peers were interpreting me as ordinary.* I needed to know whether or not they were seeing me as 'seeing.' This is why I monitored and controlled my conversations and interaction. This is why I kept an eye on social situations. It was social interaction, and this only, that could tell me whether or not I was being recognized by others as a normally seeing adolescent. It was only through social interaction that I could achieve myself, thus present myself, as such. Like everyone else, I could only be ordinary in the ordinariness of ordinary interaction.

An orientation to the other for the purposes of preserving the self is what generates anxiety. I spoke in chapter 2 of the 'fundamental anxiety' described by Schutz as an anxiety held by all of us, blind or sighted. This is the anxiety which is generated by our fundamental fear of death. The nightmare that was the story of *my* blindness during my adolescence was represented in my anxiety of being 'found out.' Being found out meant that death would come to my life of being ordinary. Since I could only be found out in an interactional situation, this death would be a slow and painful one. With few exceptions, I kept my blindness to myself.

This resulted in a death of another kind, but one much more preferable than the death of ordinary life. Nothing was more nightmarish than this, and it was a nightmare from which I could not be aroused. Waking from such a nightmare would have forced me to be awake to my difference, awake to myself as blind. I would have woken from my nightmare only to *see* my blind self being *seen* by others and would have been fully awake to the *need* to live the life of blindness. Waking up only to face such a life is something I avoided, since I did not see that life as one worth living.

This is the fundamental anxiety of adolescence. It is the anxiety of arousal and of waking to the life of difference. It is the deep sleep that precedes the arousal to the seduction of the ordinary life, of being like everyone else, and to the challenge of being like no one else, the extraordinary life.

In her discussion of the human condition, Arendt (1958, 175–6) puts the matter this way:

Human plurality, the basic condition of both action and speech, has the twofold character of equality and distinction. If men were not equal, they could neither understand each other and those who came before them nor plan for the future and foresee the needs of those who will come after them. If men were not distinct, each human being distinguished from any other who is, was, or will ever be, they would need neither speech nor action to make themselves understood.

We are simultaneously the same as, and different from, each other. From the adolescent point of view, this sameness and difference is typically understood in terms of concrete characteristics and features. Adolescent culture conceives sameness as possessing the characteristics of walking, talking, dressing, in the same way. Difference is conceived as being slightly taller or shorter than others, slightly younger or older, having blond or dark hair, and the like. This sort of sameness is desirable since it makes reference to living the ordinary life, the average life – the acceptable life. These differences make no difference whatsoever insofar as they do not point to any distinction necessitating the development of an orientation that will point *away* from sameness.

But a difference such as blindness is another story. I am not suggesting that being taller or shorter than others makes no difference to an adolescent, since if this difference is more than slight, it will make a difference. What I am suggesting is that blindness is not a difference that can be described by an adolescent, or anyone else for that matter, as slight. It is a 'marked' difference insofar as it marks and clearly distinguishes one from the other.

It is this distinction that marks blindness as a different story. Unlike a slight difference in height, blindness *demands* a story. As a distinction that makes a difference, blindness needs to be accounted for in at least two ways: first, blind persons need to provide an account of their blindness to others; and, second, they need to provide an account of it to themselves.

I am calling this account a story since blindness needs to be narrated in speech and action. It needs to be told through the living of a life. Living the life of blindness is, at the same time, telling its story. A story of blindness always-already exists in a society in a variety of collective representations. Blind persons retell these stories by the living of their lives. They may retell the story of blindness in a way that confirms collective representations or influences and modifies them. The story of blindness is told and retold in each and every instance of living the life of blindness.

Any storyteller develops an orientation both to the topic of the story and to its telling. One such orientation is that of 'adolescence.' It is this orientation that provides for the possibility of passing as the narration of blindness as a distinction that the story makes indistinguishable. But before we continue our quest to understand the adolescent orientation to blindness, let us return to the phenomenon of passing, since such a return will assist us in asking questions of the storyteller I am calling adolescence.

Let me return to passing by raising once more my concern, during my adolescence, for vigilance through monitoring interaction. Remember that I was passing as sighted, and vigilance was necessary in order to determine whether or not my speech and actions were conceived by others as those of a sighted person. I was continuously and constantly listening to the story I was telling and the reactions to it by others.

My high-school English teacher would often read aloud in class. He would often read the various plays, novels, and poems we were studying aloud to us. This reading aloud came with two requirements: first, we were required to listen; and, second, we were required to follow along in our books. The first requirement presented no difficulties to me. But the second requirement was a different story. I needed to find a way to follow along in my book without being able to see print.

As a way to find a solution to this problem, I evoked my past experiences with classroom interaction. One solution was to tell the teacher that I had forgotten my book, lost it, or, for some other reason, did not have it with me. In such cases, the teacher would ask me to move my desk alongside that of another student and to follow along in his or her book. Apart from a mild reprimand, nothing more was at stake. The beauty of this passing technique was that the other student did all of the work of 'following along,' which meant that I did not have to turn the pages, find the starting page, and the like. It had the added feature of minimizing my activity, a feature which, for anyone who passes, is conceived as a plus or, a kind of bonus, in the 'passing game.' Any time I could minimize my activities in passing, my chances of being detected as a partially sighted person were also at a minimum.

This particular strategy was not foolproof since it lacked consistency over time. Students were expected to have their books with them in class, and if on one occasion they did not, they were expected to on the next. This was a strategy which I could employ only infrequently. Frequency would have only cast suspicion upon me and raise the chances of being detected. I did what I could to be ordinary and did what I could to avoid suspicion regarding this claim. I needed to develop alternative strategies; I needed another game plan.

One such alternative involved sitting in a slouched position over my desk, a position I interpreted as acceptable male adolescent behaviour. From this position, I could more easily observe other students; thus noticing when they turned pages, I could act accordingly. But this particular method required some preparation. Turning the pages at the right time was relatively easy. The difficulty arose in finding the correct starting page since I was not able to see the pagination. I developed an alternative pagination. I made markings on every tenth page which were large enough for me to see. If we were to begin at page thirty-two, I would merely find the marking that indicated page thirty, count two more pages, and I was ready to begin confidently following along. It was important that my method of pagination was seen as such only by me. I designed it so that it would appear to others, who chanced to see it, as mere doodling.

One of the lessons I learned during this time was a lesson that many adolescents learn – the social world, with all of its phenomena, is not necessarily 'natural.' As a child, a boy is a boy, a girl is a girl, and they act in particular ways determined by the nature of gender. As an adolescent, we may learn that there are alternative ways for boys and girls to act while remaining boys and girls. We learn that boyness is not the natural fact we assumed it to be during childhood. There are alternatives, choices, and decisions to be made regarding the *kind* of boy or girl we want to be.

Along with these sorts of lessons, I learned that being sighted was not as natural as it appears. I could *be* fully sighted without *being* fully sighted.

I was recognized, interpreted, seen, and treated as fully sighted even though I was not. I accomplished all of this sightedness through ordinary interaction.

I learned more than this. I learned, through my passing, that even those who see *must* act and interact as if they can. Like me, they too had to show and display their sightedness through ordinary interaction. I came to understand that the natural fact of sightedness required the more unnatural fact of interaction. I also came to know that it was only me, in other words, only blindness, that knew this. Certainly my peers were not aware that their interaction served to display to one another that they were sighted. Their action and speech – the way they walked, the way they talked, their gestures, and even the way they dressed – pointed to the fact that they could see and that they treated the 'fact of seeing' as natural and thus took it for granted.

Their lives told the story of sightedness. In time, I came to understand this story in two ways. First, something I found surprising, I was the only one who was reading this story. I was passing as sighted, and thus knowing what sightedness 'looked like' was crucial to me. I treated my peers as though, in H.G. Wells's terms, they were citizens of the country of the sighted. To be like them, I needed to become acquainted with their customs, their ways, their language, their norms – their culture. I needed to know their story. Since their story was just there for me to read, it did not seem necessary to ask them to *tell* their story. It was also unreasonable to ask them to tell their story, given the fact they were not aware of any story being told. Asking them to do so would have certainly led to my secret stigma being divulged. In asking them to tell me their story, I would have necessarily told them mine, and my story, at least from my point of view, was not worth telling. I felt fortunate that my story was not 'just there' for them to read. My passing was my way of making my story as illegible as possible.

The second way I came to understand the story of sightedness is connected to the first. Not only was I the only one reading the story; it seemed to me, and this I found not so much surprising as I did fascinating, that I was the only one who *could* read this story. My friends and acquaintances did not know that when they were gesturing to one another that they were 'doing sight,' that they were displaying for one another that they could see. However, they were aware of such things as eye contact. They would often say, 'We made eye contact,' or 'I just stared at him,' or the like. These phrases meant getting someone's attention or showing disdain, etc. They meant the same for me, but they also meant more. These phrases also represented one of the customs, or folk-ways, of the people of the country of the sighted. This meant that I could now use these phrases and similar ones to lay claim to *my* citizenship in this country.

It was through this sort of interaction that I came to understand that my peers could not read the story of sightedness, the very story which they were telling. I came to the understanding that my peers took their sight as well as sightedness for granted. Seeing came natural to them, and, as such, it was not something they thought about or spoke about. *I came to understand that thinking about something natural required a disruption to that naturalness.* My peers could not read the story of sightedness they were telling because they could not *see* it. I understood, and understood only much later, that my blindness provided me with the 'sight' necessary to read the story of sightedness. I only recently realized that it was *me* (blindness) that was the storyteller of sightedness. (This will be developed in the final chapter.)

There is still one final lesson my passing has taught me, albeit, a lesson I learned much later. Even though sight can see much, can see shapes, colours, people's faces, newspapers, etc., *it cannot see itself.* Sight is no different from the other senses insofar as hearing cannot hear hearing, smell cannot smell smelling, and the rest. When I passed as a sighted person during my adolescence, I was recognized and treated as someone who was fully sighted. I was able to trick sight into seeing me as an instance of itself. It was as though sight, when looking at me, saw itself. It is almost like seeing *your self* in a mirror rather than its *image.* But this lesson is the lesson of adulthood insofar as it can only be learned from that standpoint. It is the same lesson gleaned from the adolescent awareness that gender is a choice, decisive, and not merely natural.

The same holds true for sightedness. Despite its physiological aspect, sightedness is not *only* natural. Typically the natural *part* of sightedness is mistaken for the *whole.* But, there is much more to sightedness and being sighted than sheer physiology. It is a social phenomenon insofar as sightedness needs to be expressed interactionally for it to be 'seen.' We inherit conceptions about sight, including the conception that sight is physiology. It is this conception that allows sight to see itself insofar as it can now 'look' at its own mechanism. Through developments in neurophysiology, sight can look at light waves emanating from physical objects and see these waves passing through the lens of the eye into the retina, through the optic nerve, and into the occipital lobe, where the retinal image is turned right side up and produces a visual image. Sight can see its mechanism and describe it. Still, sight cannot see sight. This requires thought.

Invisible, sight must be thought about, which necessitates reforming physiology into a form visible only through the sense of understanding. This is a depiction of sight and not a description.

It is this reformulation of the phenomenon of sight which brings choice into play. Every formulation of sight *could* be otherwise. Passing relies on this. It is sight understood as interactionally achievable that makes passing possible in the first place. It is sight understood as the 'paramount reality' and conceived as the normal and ordinary way-of-being which provides for any decision to pass.

From an adolescent point of view, it is better to pass and be ordinary than not. The anxiety that comes from conceiving ordinariness as the standard for living presupposes the collapse of ordinary life if the standard of ordinariness is not upheld. This was my conception of life during adolescence. I could say, with Goffman (1963, 87), that as a legally blind adolescent, I was 'living the life that' I thought could have been 'collapsed at any moment.'

Living a life that could be collapsed at any moment is certainly living precariously. This is true for all of us insofar as we are all mortal and death can collapse what we have made of ourselves at any moment. From the point of view of the adolescent who passes, life is conceived as the interactional accomplishment of ordinariness, and death is conceived as the unsuccessful accomplishment of this life.

When life is conceived as solely interaction, it flirts with death at every moment. The spirit of such a life is nothing other than anxiety and precariousness. For those who develop and maintain an adolescent relation to blindness, anxiety and precariousness are inscribed in the form of life prescribed by such a relation. Life is either held together or falls apart.

The passer comes to live a precocious life, thus learning the lessons I mentioned earlier. But this adolescent also suffers precociousness insofar as he or she comes to know, all too soon, the achieved character of social life and often cannot get past the awesomeness of its requirement. Adolescents cannot get past the awesome requirement that *they themselves* take responsibility for the making or unmaking of a reasonable and ordinary world. The adolescent comes prematurely to the responsibility of making a life and holding it together.

The adolescent understands interaction as the way to secure a life. This adolescent copies what he or she conceives as *real* and *natural* and through this copying achieves him- or herself as such. The *realness* of *life* is ruled by the standards of normalcy and ordinariness. This is why the passer's life is so precarious and so anxiety-riddled. The ordinary life *fears* extraordinariness and *trembles* at its possibility and *falls* before its appearance. Passing is not restricted to blind adolescents. Such activities are the domain of adolescence *per se*. Passing is often understood under the rubric of socialization. Adolescence is often understood as the copying of adulthood and as the last step toward it. An adolescent engaged in smoking, drinking, and sex is understood as expressing the desire for adulthood. 'Sex, drugs, and rock and roll,' on the other hand, is often understood as an expression of the lack of desire for adulthood. But adolescence sees this as the desire to re-form adulthood. Regardless of particular conceptions and understandings, however, the copying of adulthood by adolescents is understood as progress insofar as it expresses a move from adolescence.

The blind adolescent who passes as sighted may be understood in a similar way. Passing is the expression of knowing the sighted nature of the social world as well as a desire to interact in that world as simply another citizen. It is the desire to live life as a person who 'happens to be blind.' But the living of such a life requires the adolescent to mature by recognizing the limits of a life dedicated to copying. The adolescent must come to understand that *any* life ruled by the standards of normalcy and ordinariness is necessarily emptied of *any* significance or value. The adolescent must come to understand the relation between his or her own orientation to normalcy and ordinariness, and the 'shadowy' unauthentic life that results.

But this maturing is easier said than done. To the adolescent, any version of limit is itself limited in that it is conceived negatively. Any limit attached to the life of copying expresses nothing other than the undesirable death of ordinary life. Such a death comes to the adolescent when she or he is 'found out,' *found* to be blind. The life of blindness represents a stigmatizing mark that must be lived with, and such a life is not worth living, for it would only point to and highlight what it lacks and how it fails.

To think of blindness in this way certainly represents alienation. Its animus is ordinariness, and its focus is on ordinariness conceived as an achievable standard. This life casts its difference aside by hiding it, thus favouring and privileging the life of ordinariness by displaying it. It hides blindness under the cover of sightedness by interactionally constructing sight as a superficial cloak. This life hides its blindness not only from others but also *from itself*. It alienates itself from itself.

It is no wonder that passing is fraught with anxiety. This anxiety finds its possibility in ordinariness conceived as a standard for the 'good life' since, as such, ordinariness privileges sameness and ignores difference, thus making it vulnerable to inevitable collapse much in the same way that the mountain of security surrounding the country of the blind collapsed. Living ordinary life *as if* it were the whole of life is, without question, the nightmarish terror of self-alienation. In his short story 'The Death of Ivan Ilyich,' Tolstoy (1978, 109) writes, 'Ivan Ilyich's life had been most simple and most ordinary and therefore most terrible.' If a most ordinary life is a most terrible life, then the life that desperately desires to be most ordinary must be the most terrible life of all. It is one thing to live ordinarily with ordinary conditions and quite another to do so with the extraordinary condition of blindness.

Blindness does not permit a life taken for granted in the way that sightedness does, and blindness *especially* does not permit taking sightedness for granted. Everything falls away and disappears in the face of blindness. Blind persons cannot simply 'look and see,' and thus they must be consciously aware of both their physical and social environment as they move about the world. Contrary to rehabilitation's view, doing ordinary things is not itself an ordinary thing for blind persons.

If the living of an ordinary life is conceived as the greatest possible achievement, the highest good, and the ultimate end of life, then blind persons who adopt this conception are forced to continuously and constantly orient to ordinariness as the standard of their lives. This orientation is what generates the need for blind persons to pass as sighted. This commitment is at one and the same time a commitment to self-alienation and the subsequent terrible life of anxiety. Taking liberties with Tolstoy's words, 'His artful passing had made his life most natural and most ordinary and, therefore, most terrible.'

It is this terror that signifies the limits of passing. The adolescent *must* come to recognize these limits if a more adult orientation to blindness is to be developed. So far the examples of passing I have made use of do not recognize any version of its limits. These examples display deception as an essential feature of passing. As a way to address its limits, I want now to provide examples of passing that do not display deception as one of its essential features.

I often attend sports events such as ice hockey games with friends who are aware that I am a legally blind person. About my blindness, in particular how it relates to attending ice hockey games, my friends know what I know. They know that I am not able to distinguish one player from another. They know, too, that I cannot see the puck. Both my friends and I know that I am not able to watch the game in the way everyone else does and, therefore, I must make use of other means as a way to understand what is happening during the course of the game. I am unable to see whether or not a goal has been scored.

But there are other occurrences during a game that I make use of as a way to know whether a goal has been scored. (Let me say that sighted persons do the same thing.) In some instances, when a goal has been scored there is a loud noise that occurs when the frozen rubber puck hits the metal portions of the goal net. But in and of itself, this noise does not signify, with any guarantee, that a goal has been scored since the noise could have been caused by the puck hitting the outside frame of the net. If this noise is accompanied by a loud cheer, I can be almost certain that a goal has been scored by the home team. Or, if this noise is accompanied by a relative silence in the arena together with less frenzied action on the ice, I can be as certain that the opposing team has scored.

These and many other indications allow me to react appropriately to a goal being scored or to other relevant events that happen during the course of the game. If I happen to miss one of these events, my friends will describe it to me. The point is that I am able to orient to activities which allow me to act and interact appropriately at a hockey game. It is important to note here that there may be occasions that my friends, or any other of the spectators for that matter, themselves do not see a goal being scored and thus use the very same indications that I do to recognize the goal. It is not relevant that my friends see the puck go into the net since they can claim that they either saw it or did not. I, on the other hand, can only and always make the latter claim. Still, I respond to a goal being scored in the same way that my friends and other spectators do. This response interactionally makes the claim that I have seen the puck go into the net or, at least, could have.

Even though the other spectators are not aware of my legal blindness, my friends certainly are and, despite my response to a goal being scored, know that I neither saw the puck go into the net nor could I have seen it do so. My friends recognize my response to a goal being scored and treat it as legitimate. They do not chide me for cheering, and since they already know I am legally blind, they do not use my cheering as an occasion to topicalize it. This does not seem to be living a life that could collapse at any moment. Part of the reason for this is that there is no deception involved. My friends know that I am legally blind and know that I cannot watch the hockey game. But they also know that I enjoy attending hockey games and that there are ways, for all practical purposes, for me to know what is occurring. As one of my friends once put it, 'Yah, he's got ways, he knows what's going on.'

There are still other occasions when being found out does not result in any collapse of life. During conversations, I attempt to make what citizens of the country of the sighted call 'eye contact.' This presents some difficulty to me. My central vision is blocked out, and I have only a little peripheral vision. In order to see the face of the person with whom I am speaking, I must move this blocked-out area out of the way and look around it. When I see people's faces, it will appear to them as though I am looking past them. From my point of view, I am actually looking at them. Now if I am successful in focusing this blocked-out area on people's faces, it will appear to them as though I am looking into their eyes or at least into their faces. For me, making eye contact has nothing to do with seeing. When I see a person's face, I know that I am not looking into it, and when I do not see the face, I know that that is where I am looking. When I am unsuccessful in this procedure or when I explain it to others, neither interactional collapse nor disaster occurs.

So far I have described two situations in which I pass: first, there is the situation in which no one knows, except me, that I am legally blind; second, there is the situation in which others know. In the latter situation, my intention is not to deceive anyone but to demonstrate to them, as well as to myself, that I am able to orient both to the sightedness of others and to the pragmatic requirements of a 'sighted world.' This signifies a development from the first type of passing insofar as deception is no longer a key feature.

Here is another example of such passing. Before I arrived at the university at which I conducted my graduate work, I telephoned and wrote letters to many of the professors telling them about my legal blindness. Upon arriving at the university, I met with professors and spoke extensively about my blindness, especially since I was planning to conduct my graduate research on that topic. I also spoke about my blindness with many of the graduate students.

My partial sightedness did not permit me to recognize people simply by looking at their faces. I made use of other indicators as a means to recognize them – indicators such as height, weight, style of dress, typical posture in standing, walking, as well as many other features, such as style and colour of hair, whether or not they had beards, wore glasses, and so on. The most important indicator was voice.

It takes time to more or less successfully recognize people on the basis of such indicators. It takes time to determine a person's typical posture or typical style of dress. In order to recognize people, I always tried to glean as much of this sort of information as possible. Until then, I made use of other procedures in order to demonstrate that I *should* be able to recognize people in a certain social setting. When my professors or fellow graduate students greeted me with a 'good morning' or a 'hello' during the first few weeks at the university, I did not typically respond to their greetings in the same way. Instead, I responded in such a way so as to maximize the possibility of their speaking again. I would respond, for example, with a 'Hello, how are you?' This return greeting is also a question and would typically elicit more talk. They would typically respond with a 'fine' or an 'OK,' or the like. This extra bit of talk would allow me to make a more positive identification and would allow me to become more familiar with their voices.

A feature of any social setting is the people who make it up. A university setting is made up largely of professors and students. Being familiar with a social setting is another procedure for recognizing people. In time, I come to know who I can expect to see in a particular setting since those present are usually connected to it. In a setting to which I am connected, I operate with the assumption that I should know and thus recognize other members of that setting. As such, I treat these people as people to whom I am interactionally committed insofar as we share the same social setting. I assume these people share a similar commitment.

Such an assumption means that I operate with the expectation that others will greet me in this shared setting and that they expect the same of me. One of the characteristics of the university department I worked in was a long hallway with offices and other rooms on either side. When I walked down this hallway, I often noticed someone walking toward me from the other end. I did not visually notice them, since my noticing was done largely through hearing and some perception of shadows. The distance between us made it impossible for me to recognize who was walking my way. *Anyone* in that setting was treated by me as someone who belonged there and thus as someone to whom I was interactionally committed. A greeting from both of us was something I understood as an interactional expectation. If a greeting was not forthcoming from either of us, this would have to be made sense of in one way or another. One way to make sense of this would be to interpret someone in such a situation as a 'snob' or, at least, as someone who was 'snubbing.'[2] Not wanting to be interpreted in this way, I would always greet a person in this situation.

2 Turner (1974, 197–215) provides an excellent analysis of 'snubs' and their interactional achievement and use. McHugh et al. (1974, 109–36) address the 'grammar' of 'snubs' and display the social auspices under which they operate.

But I would never wait for the other person to greet me first. I would always initiate the greeting, thus providing the other the opportunity, in fact, obligation to greet me in return. In this way, I prevented any interpretation of me snubbing anyone. The two of us were in the same setting, and I initiated a greeting.

This solution was not without its risks. Despite the fact that I interpreted the person at the other end of the hallway as being interactionally committed to the setting, as being a professor, another graduate student, a clerical worker, or the like, the possibility still existed that the person may have been a stranger. The person at the other end of the hallway could well have questioned the interactional appropriateness of my greeting. Greeting someone we do not know and who does not know us is often treated with suspicion. Someone who greets strangers is sometimes considered to be a very cheerful person or, at other times, a 'nut.'

Thus to minimize this interpretation, especially the latter, I made use of the more appropriate non-verbal greeting. I often made use of the 'smile.' The smile is interesting in many ways insofar as it reveals many things. Most important to me, at that time, was how the smile functioned. A smile could function as a greeting between acquaintances or, simply, as an acknowledgment of another. Smiling at a stranger on a crowded city sidewalk may raise suspicion, but two strangers smiling at each other in an otherwise unoccupied hallway is appropriate. A smile was not only an interactionally appropriate greeting but also less risky than a more friendly verbal greeting. If the person at the other end of the hallway verbally greeted me first, then my interactional problem was non-existent.

The smile is particularly useful in passing as well as in demonstrating interactional competence. Whenever I left, or returned to, my residence at the university, I passed by my neighbour's kitchen window. My neighbour was a friend and knew of my legal blindness. When his kitchen window was open and he was standing at it as I walked by, he would call out a greeting or, if the window was closed, he would simply wave. When he called out a greeting, I knew that he was standing at the window and thus returned his greeting. When he did not call out, I did not know whether or not he was standing at his window waving.

I once again resorted to the smile. When I passed by my neighbour's window and received no verbal greeting, I simply looked toward the window and smiled. This took care of two things; I initiated a greeting, and, if my neighbour was at his window waving at me, I returned his greeting. Instead of smiling, I could have waved. This would have been fine if my neighbour was at his window. But, since I was not sure of this, a wave, particularly at no one, would have looked 'silly' to those who may have happened to see me doing so. The smile was interactionally safer. Even if someone had seen me smiling, and smiling at no one, they could have interpreted me as someone in a good mood or as someone who had just thought of something amusing.

Much of my passing is conducted in settings to which I am not interactionally committed – settings such as large office buildings, public transportation, and city streets. In these settings, it is important to me, as it is to everyone, that actions are seen as sensible and ordinary. It is important that my actions are seen as such 'at first glance.'[3] All of us know and take for granted that, when in a public setting, we are visually available to others. Others can see us. Typically, all of us want to influence *how* we are seen in public places. We want others to see us as people who are normal, ordinary members of a public setting. All of us engage in interactional work to maximize the possibility of being seen as such. Such work is almost always taken for granted by persons who can see; thus they do not typically *see* the sort of work they do. Those who are blind *see* this work, and see it only too well.

I am aware of this interactional work and aware too that I must consciously 'do' this work in order to display my *bona fide* membership in a culture. This display means that I must interactionally influence others to see me, and do so at a glance, as a *bona fide* sighted member of a culture. Influencing people in this way is not animated by a sense of deception. I am not attempting to deceive people in a public place.

During my graduate school years I had enough residual vision to 'get around' without using a white cane or a dog guide. I carried no mark or symbol of blindness. There were only two ways that the crowds of people in a public place would know that I was legally blind. One way was for me to simply tell them. Another was for them to interpret me as such by seeing me fall down a flight of stairs, walk into something, or the like. Either way was not acceptable. It would have been extremely unusual for me to announce to a mass of people that I was legally blind. Falling down stairs, or the like, may have led to interpretations other than blindness, such as inattentiveness or drunkenness. Neither way was reasonable to me. Still, not telling people in a public place that I was legally blind had nothing to do with deception. It was no more deceiving than not telling them that I was a graduate student, or that I was married, or some such thing.

Many blind persons, whether they have residual sight or not, pass as

3 For an analysis of the 'glance' in everyday interaction, see Sudnow 1972.

sighted. They pass, not to deceive others into thinking that they are sighted, but to display to others that they recognize the sighted character of the world and that they are able to fit in. This sort of passing, unlike sheer adolescent passing animated by deception, aims to display to others an intimacy with sight. This sort of passing may be understood as a solution to the problem we raised in the last chapter, the problem of the privatization of blindness.

This particular solution orients to sightedness as the normal-state-of-affairs. It orients to sightedness as providing the *only* possibility for the common experience of public life. Passing conceives of blindness as a lack, but not merely as the lack of the physiological ability to see. It conceives blindness as lacking something more than this. It sees blindness as lacking common experience, as lacking the essential feature of seeing a world in common. It is this lack to which passing is oriented and which, in turn, orients passing. Passing is posed as a solution to the problem of lack insofar as it aims to demonstrate that blindness can coexist in a world where sightedness is essential. It seeks to display that blindness can shadow sight and can thus share a world-in-common.

This sort of passer is resisting any temptation to be characterized solely on the basis of blindness. Passing is more than the sheer instrumentality of surviving in a sighted world. Passing teaches the blind person that he or she must display a regard for sightedness in the presentation of who he or she is and thus resist the temptation to understand him- or herself and the world shared with others through 'blind eyes' alone. Persons who see must also invent a way to display their regard for blind persons if the two groups are to cohabit a world in a way that is not merely some weak version of multiculturalism. For, where a culture expresses itself without regard for difference, it cuts off anyone and anything different as a speaker with something to bring to it, with something to teach it about itself, and this means that only the most distal and technical kind of exchange of information will be able to occur between them. Even if sightedness displays itself without a regard for blindness, as it often does, blindness can never do the same. Passing (surviving) in a sighted world requires that the blind person learn to display his or her regard for sightedness as essential to his or her expression and definition of who he or she is.

All of this points to the understanding that, from the point of view of blindness, the world is sighted. In order for a blind person to carry on any activity in the world she or he must orient to that world as sighted. Blind persons know that their activities in the world are visually available to others. They know that they are observable. In this regard, there is no difference between someone who can see and someone who cannot. Both must live in a world where life, at least its public aspect, is observable to others. Insofar as the life of sightedness takes this for granted, the life of blindness acts as teacher. Blindness can remind sightedness of what it *sees* but typically does not look at.

Through an examination of passing we are beginning to see the possibility of a relationship between blindness and sightedness that goes beyond the one established by Nunez and the citizens of the country of the blind. Nunez represented enlightenment, and the citizens of the country of the blind represented ignorance. Such a relation allows for only *one* teacher. From his view, a view endowed with the natural fortune of sightedness, Nunez had much to teach the citizens. Other than the natural endowment of the human ability to adapt to any condition, even blindness, Nunez had nothing to learn from blindness.

We are beginning now to grasp a richer sense of what I meant by the 'adolescent' relation to blindness. This relation holds blindness as secondary to sightedness much in the same way that adolescence is secondary to adulthood. In the conventional conception of adolescence as a temporary stage and as the step toward adulthood, adolescence is understood as 'incomplete.'[4] It is so insofar as adulthood is conceived as the maturation stage of the life-cycle. This view characterizes adolescence as immature insofar as it is on-the-way-to ... and thus not yet completely adult.

The eyes of a newborn are understood in a similar way. These eyes are not yet physiologically fully formed, and thus the newborn is not yet able to see. The ability to see requires two things: first, it requires the physiological maturation of eyes; and, second, it requires an upbringing which teaches the newborn what there is to see and how to look at it. A newborn's sight is incomplete and immature. But, a newborn is on the way to seeing.

The onset of blindness, regardless of the chronological age at which it occurs, puts a stop to this maturation process. Unlike the eyes of a newborn, blind eyes are *not* on their way to seeing. These eyes are *essentially* incomplete. They can come to know that there is seeing, but they can never see. These eyes can come *close* to maturity, but they can never *be* mature.

It is this understanding of seeing and sight that gives birth to the development of an adolescent relation to blindness. Blindness is always-already

---

4 Elsewhere (1984, 296–311), I argue for the 'completeness' of adolescence.

immature in relation to the maturity of sightedness. 'Mature blindness' is conceived as coming close, or shadowing, sightedness. The only hope held out for blindness is that it will reach adolescence and come close to the maturity of adulthood.

It is no wonder that the adoption and development of an adolescent relation to blindness is so tempting, and is so not only to blind persons but also to persons who see. In the face of blindness conceived as lack, and as unnatural and incomplete, it is tempting to at least come close to that which is complete – to come close to sightedness. It is tempting to succumb to the beckoning seduction of sightedness, wrapped, as it is, in the social cloak of the promise of intimacy with completion and maturity. Living the adolescent life of blindness means that the blind person has been seduced by sight's conception of itself as the most mature, most complete, most ordinary, most natural, and therefore most enjoyable life. This most enjoyable life is, however, not a life that can be lived by a blind person. It is a life that a blind person can only cling to, only shadow, can only be infatuated with. It is a life that is seductive and, as such, is a life that is forever and always steeped in mystery. The seducer, in order to remain seductive, must always remain mysterious and ever so slightly out of grasp.

But blindness is never a mystery. No one is ever infatuated with it. There is nothing seductive about blindness, and this is why adolescence never chooses it as a decisive way to live. Adolescence rejects blindness in favour of the mysterious life of sightedness, a life it can only shadow.

Blindness can never hold itself up, in the face of sightedness, as a choice-worthy life. Blindness is always conceived as a *condition* that must be lived with. No one conceives of themselves as living with the condition of sight. Those who see, 'see themselves' as *seeing*. Sighted persons are never spoken of as 'persons who happen to be sighted.' No sighted person, in the history of personhood, has ever been chided for not 'accepting' his or her sightedness. At most, 'Watch where you're going!' is an admonishment sometimes given.

Blindness is lived with only 'when all else fails,' which means when all attempts to banish the condition by restoring sight, fail. It is under these auspices that the adolescent relation to blindness functions and invents passing as a method for ridding the self of the condition of blindness. This is how ophthalmology and rehabilitation can both be committed to 'sight restoration.' The one restores it through the practices of medicine, while the other does so through the practice of imparting techniques for the 'activities of daily living.' Regardless of their individual differences, both disciplines orient to sightedness as completeness and hence the standard for *any* life of blindness.

One final word on adolescence – a word we leave for Erikson to speak since, even today, he is considered to be the quintessential expert on the human maturation process and thus on adolescence:

As technological advances put more and more time between early school life and the young person's final access to specialized work, the stage of adolescing becomes an even more marked and conscious period and, as it has always been in some cultures in some periods, almost a way of life between childhood and adulthood. Thus in the later school years young people, beset with the physiological revolution of their genital maturation and the uncertainty of the adult roles ahead, seem much concerned with faddish attempts at establishing an adolescent subculture with what looks like a final rather than a transitory or, in fact, initial identity formation. (Erikson 1968, 128)

In speaking about the 'concerned' adolescent, Erikson speaks about his own concern, a concern which, remember, is spoken from the point of view of an adult. We might even say that Erikson represents the 'concerns' of adulthood as they relate to adolescence. This adult concern, in Erikson's view, stems from 'technological advances,' advances, we might add, advanced by adults. Nonetheless, the concern is that technological advances have widened the gap between 'early school life' (Erikson's term for childhood) and 'specialized work' (his term for adulthood).

But the concern goes even further than this. This ever-widening gap between childhood and adulthood, the gap called adolescence, means that adolescents are such for a longer period of time. Like any other 'gap of time,' this one too shall be filled. The concern of adulthood is that it will be filled by adolescence. The concern is that adolescents will make of their time what they will. Left to their own devices, who knows what they will make?[5] This is an adult concern with adolescence, and it is especially concerning since, as Scholl and Holman (1981, 72) tell us, 'Adolescence is a transitional stage between the security of the child and the yet unknown world of the adult.' The adolescent resides in the gap between security and certainty. No wonder that adolescence is such a tumultuous

---

5 In this sense, Erikson acts more like a babysitter than a scholar. He seems to continually watch over adolescents with the particular aim of examining what they make and making sure that this making conforms to the adult version of what *should* be made in this gap he calls 'adolescing.'

time, and no wonder adults are so concerned with it. Who knows what those who are neither secure nor certain will make?

Erikson's concern is that adolescence will make something permanent and final out of what is essentially temporary and incomplete. We can see how such a concern, on the part of adulthood, comes about. The adolescent, missing the security of childhood and facing the yet unknown realm of adulthood, is tempted to treat his or her position in this gap as if it were permanent and final. Adolescence creates fads and treats them as if they were the customs and norms of a permanent culture, rather than the fleeting fads of a temporary subculture. Adolescents act as adolescents are wont to do, impatiently, and through this impatience create their life-world as if it were the finality of adulthood rather than the final step toward it.

The adoption of an adolescent relation to blindness stems from a similar concern to that of Erikson, but with an interesting ironic twist. Blindness is concerned, not with conceiving itself as temporary, as adolescence does, but rather it concerns itself with finality and permanence. Any person who loses their sight hopes desperately that blindness is not final. He or she hopes that blindness is a temporary and not a permanent condition. Thus living with blindness with *finality* is, for many blind persons, living with sightedness as the 'paramount reality' and thus living a life committed to adapting in a sighted world. Sightedness is a permanent thing, whereas blindness is an anomaly, and, like any anomaly, it comes and goes. Even when blindness comes and stays, many of us live in a way that does not treat it as final. The 'final word' on reality – its nature, its essence, etc. – is the word spoken by sightedness and not by blindness. *This is why no blind person ever believes what they see.*

Whatever truth lies in all of this, blind persons *must* and do live with blindness, and live with it in particular ways. One such way, a way I have tried to speak about in this chapter, is the adolescent way. This way of living with blindness provides for the possibility of passing as sighted and is thereby steeped in deception. Deception is clearly manifested in those blind persons who act *as if* they can see. But it is also present, albeit in a more blurry sense, in those blind persons who act *as if* what they see cannot possibly be real. In this latter case, the 'as if' is not an essential part of the activity of passing. Most of us who are blind know that what we see is not real and thus do not have to act as if it were. Nonetheless, our reality is different from most. It is this reality of this 'most' that we typically understand as the real perception.

It is in this way that the adolescent relation to blindness commits itself

to sightedness as the 'final word.' Passing becomes a way for blind persons to live a life which displays their hearing, and believing, of this word.
This commitment makes it difficult, if not impossible, to hear the word of
blindness over the 'noise of sightedness.' The difficulty, for both blind
and sighted persons, lies in conceiving blindness as having something to
say in a world understood as sighted. This problem, however, comes only
with the development of a more mature relation to blindness.

I have already hinted at such a relation by raising the possibility of
blindness being conceived as teacher. To this possibility rehabilitation
has nothing more to say. Rehabilitation involves itself in training blind
persons, and rightly so. All of us, blind or sighted, require training in the
technical aspects of life. But if we are to allow our life to teach us, we must
begin to understand that life as teacher. We must begin to *hear* the voice
of the teacher that resonates with blindness. It is this voice that is the next
speaker in our story.

6

The Shadow of Blindness

We began our story of blindness with its discovery and diagnosis, where we saw how forcefully blindness influenced the life of a person. So forceful was this influence that it overwhelmed any and every sense of reality for the newly blinded person or any sense of expectations for the parents of a blind offspring. Blindness shattered the assumptions that, until its onset, were held securely in the grasp of a world taken for granted. We then saw how ophthalmology acted as the final arbiter in judging, through its diagnostic practices, whether or not blindness would be a permanent feature of a person's life. Rehabilitation entered the story of blindness at this point as an actor committed to influencing the forcefulness of blindness by minimizing its overwhelming effects through imparting a set of techniques for carrying on the activities of daily life. We saw, finally, through the example of blind adolescence, how it is necessary for a blind person to develop some relation to blindness and to think about it in one way or another.

All of this I have called the 'story of blindness,' and all of the particularities, such as discovery, diagnosis, ophthalmology, etc., I have called the voices and tellers of this story. Every one of these voices has its own particular story to tell. The voice of discovery tells the story of 'terror' in that it tells of how blindness terrorizes the security that sight brings to the world in a taken-for-granted way. It tells of how this terrorist may strike, and may strike anyone, at any time and at any place.

The voice of ophthalmology, in contrast, brings the voice of 'reason' to the story of blindness insofar as it inserts a reasonable medical account. But ophthalmology tells its story with two voices; it speaks either with the voice of joy or of gloom. It brings joy when sight restoration is possible, and, when it is not, ophthalmology brings the voice of gloom.

Rehabilitation enters this story almost as forcefully as does blindness and enters it with the determined voice of practicality and will. In its telling, rehabilitation voices the practical determination and strong-willed character of personhood and speaks of how the 'person' can influence and overcome any condition, including blindness. Rehabilitation gives voice to the 'practical fact' that, despite its force, blindness cannot forcefully remove the 'person' from the blind person, and thus the person, even as blind, remains like anyone else and like she or he always was, an 'ordinary person' sharing in the determined practicality and will of personhood.

Then adolescence speaks, and, like the others, it speaks in the midst of this on-going conversation which is the story of blindness. It seems, though, to single out the voice of personhood and to speak directly to it. Adolescence speaks with the desperate voice of anxiety and tries to tell the voice of personhood that despite how practically determined and wilful it is, its reinsertion into blindness is fraught with anxiety. Adolescence speaks of the power and beauty of sight and how, as such, sight would *never* desire to live together with the brutish ugliness of blindness. At best, sight would permit, sometimes graciously and sometimes not, blindness to inhabit its world, but it would *never ever* enter into the mutually respectful and admiring life of cohabitation. But because adolescence is infatuated with the powerful and beautiful world of seeing, it desperately seeks any chance for such cohabitation. The only chance that adolescence can imagine for the fulfilment of its desire to become powerful and beautiful is 'deception.' Adolescent blindness must deceive sightedness, as well as itself, into thinking that it is also powerful and beautiful. It must live deceptively, acting *as if* it, too, can see. When adolescence tells its side of the story of blindness, it does so with the voice of anxiety.

Into this conversation, which sometimes exhibits clarity, at other times confusion, and still at other times contradiction, enters the voice of adulthood. As was the case for adolescence, I am not using the term 'adulthood' in a strictly chronological sense. Now it may turn out during the course of these deliberations that I do use this term in correspondence with an age that we typically conceive of as 'adult,' but, for the most part, my intention is to use it to make reference to the idea of 'maturity'; thus, I use 'adulthood' metaphorically. Maturity does not signify some ontological form of human existence. Instead, I make use of this term in a relational sense that seeks to represent how we relate to blindness, how we think of it, and how we conceive it. I devote this chapter to an attempt to develop a mature relation to blindness which seeks to privilege neither personhood nor the force of condition, but which aims at integrating the two; and which represents blindness, first of all, as a life and, second, as a life worth living. But we are not yet done with passing since the path to maturity, which may be the very thing we call maturity, represents a journey upon which passing has a place. I want to begin our path to maturity by reintroducing the passer.

Remember that the adolescent passer treated passing as a method for deception. The adolescent was interested primarily in presenting a self in such a way that this self would be interpreted, in a taken-for-granted way, as a 'seeing self.' 'Seeing' coursed through the very being of the adolescent. The adolescent not only presented him- or herself as a 'seeing self' to others but presented this *same* self to him- or herself. He or she thought of the self and felt the self to be, through and through, a self who sees.

Even though I was legally blind, recall that I had *some* residual vision. This meant that I was more effective at passing than I would have been had I none. But it meant something else as well: my sense of self was wrapped tightly in an identity defined by me as nothing other than seeing, and this, despite the fact that my sight was severely limited and what sight I had was slowly, yet noticeably, slipping away. As my sight slipped away, so did my identity. What I was *really* losing, then, when I was 'losing my sight,' and perhaps this is true for everyone who goes blind, was my sense of self.

This allows me to cast the idea of passing, and the need for it, in a different light. My need for passing was born of my need to present myself as sighted, and my conception of passing was that it was strictly and only a method for doing so and that it was the only method available. I needed to present myself as sighted, and the only way to do so was to act as if I were. I clung fast to my limited residual sight and did so as if it were full sight and not partial. I also loosened my grip on blindness and let it slip away as suddenly as it came and as quickly as my residual sight was slipping. In clinging to my residual sight, I was at the same time clinging to what was left of myself. As my sight slipped away, so did my self, and the more it slipped, the more fast I clung to it.

But blindness proved to be as stubborn as I was. It clung to me with a grip as strong as the one I had on sightedness. 'Caught in the grip of blindness' was how I understood my fate during adolescence. I could not escape blindness no matter what I did, and what I did was pass as sighted, something I understood as being *forced* upon me by blindness. Passing was my way of inserting my self into the social world in the face of the deplorable condition of blindness. Ophthalmology could not banish this condition from my life – it had nothing more to say or do – and so I took matters into my own hands and decided to overpower the force of blindness with my sighted self.

The more I passed, which is another way of saying the older I grew and the more sight I lost, the more difficult and the more anxiety-riddled my life became. This meant, simply, that deceiving others into thinking that I was sighted became arduous, and thus the level of my anxiety was raised. It was almost as though blindness and sightedness were in the throes of a battle, with my self going to the victor, and it seemed that blindness was winning. My whole life was involved in developing and implementing strategies to stave off the attacks of blindness, thus maintaining my presentation of self as a 'seeing self.'

Being *both* blind and sighted, having a 'mixed nature,' was not within the realm of my self-identity possibilities. I had to be one or the other. I could not be both. Being both would have been like being alive and dead at the same time. It seemed to me that being both sighted and blind was impossible since the two were opposite to each other and opposed to one another and the latter was antithetical to the former. The two natures could not be mixed and thus could not be integrated into wholeness. It was *either* one *or* the other but not *both*.

Such an understanding of the co-presence of blindness and sightedness is derivative insofar as it stems from some unified conception of both. Conceiving of blindness and sightedness as opposed to one another meant that I held some assumptions and presuppositions about the two. Passing as sighted meant that I conceived of sight as the way life should be, as the natural order of things, as normal, thus first, as thesis. That I thought of blindness as opposite to sight meant that it was opposite to all that sight was, to all that it stood for and represented. Sight was normal and natural and, as such, should be counted on and presupposed as the natural way of being-in-the-world. Everyone who was, is, or ever will be, was, is, and will be *sighted*. Everyone was a person, a person in the way everyone else was a person, and everyone was an ordinary person. Everything out of the ordinary in relation to personhood would come from something extra to this ordinariness. Persons could be extraordinarily attractive, or extraordinarily strong, or extraordinarily musical, or extraordinarily intelligent. Ordinary persons may become extraordinary through outstanding achievements in scholastics or athletics, or through the acquisition of wealth or fame, etc. But all which is extraordinary is an embellishment, an exaggeration, or, better, an enhancement of that which is ordinary. This is why extraordinary people can always legitimately claim ordinariness, and why ordinary people can always relate to those who are extraordinary. Thus, the disablist adage 'As famous as he is, he still puts on his pants one leg at a time, just like me.'

But there is still another way of becoming extraordinary which is *not* an embellishment of what is ordinary. Disability, in whatever form it takes and as extraordinary as it may be, is typically understood as a 'corruption' of that which is ordinary and not as an embellishment. Unlike the ordinary way of becoming extraordinary, this way is never applauded. We do whatever we can to prevent becoming extraordinary in this way; hence, as I said in chapter 2, the development of prevention-of-blindness programs.

It is in these ways that, as an adolescent, I conceived the relation between blindness and sightedness. Blindness was opposite to sight because it lacked an essential feature of personhood and because it was a corruption of sight. It was a form of extraordinariness which I neither valued nor desired. At that time, and this has not significantly changed, my society did not present 'positive' conceptions or collective representations of blindness. The opposite was the case. Since I did not possess any extraordinary musical ability, something which is often assumed blind persons do possess, I thought my future career would consist, and I mean this quite literally, of selling pencils on a street corner or working in a broom factory. But what was most important to me was that blindness meant I could no longer be 'one of the guys.'

My decision to pass as sighted derived from a prior decision. Passing was grounded in how I chose to understand my choices for being-in-the-world. My understanding was that I could be *either* blind *or* sighted but not *both*. Since choosing blindness would be choosing what was opposite to sight and thus antithetical to everything normal and natural, I chose sightedness.

This is where what I have called 'adolescent passing' finds its possibility. This means that even though blindness and sightedness can be co-present, they can never coexist. They can live side by side, but never together. An adolescent relation to blindness does not permit for blindness and sightedness to live together in a society *or* in an individual. Blindness can only come *close* to sightedness, but it can never *touch* it. Faced with the choice, everyone would and would always choose sightedness.

From this point of view, the world is truly sighted. As such, blind persons must try to 'fit in.' Making a place or even finding a place is impossible for blindness since there *is* no place for it in the sighted world. At best, the sighted world will allow blindness to 'fit in' and even 'fit it in.'

The sighted world will *accommodate* blindness. The best this world can do is to develop a 'charitable tolerance' for blindness. The best a blind person can do is to display the adaptability of personhood by 'fitting into' the sighted world. The choice becomes to 'fight and fight and fight' through passing as sighted or to 'fight and fight and fight' for the privilege of fitting in.

Fitting in, however, is a more mature way of addressing blindness than is passing. But both ways understand 'adaptation' as the answer to the question What is blindness? Both see technique, either techniques for passing or techniques for fitting in, as the solution to the problem of blindness. Harking back to Kierkegaard's 'man,' the problem of blindness has been raised, solved, and done with. Any search for blindness is now replaced by a search for technique. The question of blindness has been answered and no longer needs to be asked. Harking back to Heidegger, this is what is most 'thought-provoking.'

But if we listen more carefully to passing and to the desire for fitting in, we may hear something more than technique. However, we must not allow ourselves to be tempted by the amazing character of technology and thus distracted by its feats. To use an analogy, we must go beyond being amazed that people can now travel in space and listen to what this can teach us. We must go beyond the amazing techniques for adapting, for fitting in, and even for passing and listen to what *this* can teach us. Let us once again ask the question What can blindness teach us?

This means that we must orient to blindness as *teacher*. Indeed, we may have been doing so all along. Blindness has taught us and reminded us, yet once again, of our overriding respect for adaptation and our fundamental commitment to personhood. We are reminded that, no matter what happens to us, personhood together with its salient feature of adaptation will 'pull us through.' We are reminded of, what some have called, the 'human spirit.'[1] To learn this, we must treat blindness as 'adversity' and, in the face of it, be reminded of the strength of the human spirit.

There is a valuable lesson to be learned from this form of humanism. It teaches us, and this may be its most valuable lesson, that blindness can, *in fact,* be lived with. Despite all the social-psychological as well as physical turmoil blindness brings, the human spirit will win out. The human spirit

---

1 Perhaps the most articulate expression of this form of humanism comes from Frankl (1969). Here Frankl speaks of the strength of the human spirit in the face of the most horrific of all human conditions, namely, the Holocaust and its companion 'death camps.'

can overcome all and any adversity. This form of humanism treats adversity as an occasion for the human spirit to show itself through a dramatic display of strength.

The question now is whether or not there is anything else to be learned from blindness. Is it just another form of adversity? Is blindness just one more condition, among many, to which we must adapt? Does blindness possess a power different from any other negative condition? Is it yet one more occasion for us to say, 'Life goes on'? Does blindness represent a valid way of seeing or only the invalidity that comes from a distortion?

Questions such as these are raised by the 'story of blindness' told as the story of human adaptation to negative conditions. They are not asked in the polemic spirit of questioning the validity of such a story. On the contrary, such questions reconfirm the story of adaptation as valid insofar as they ask whether or not there is something else that blindness can show us and teach us. Along with asking, these questions also *say* something. They say that there *is* something particular that blindness teaches us about human adaptation and the human spirit. These questions ask whether blindness can teach us something else, and they ask whether there is something *more* to blindness than the lesson of the power of human adaptation. These questions say that the story of human adaptation is *part* of the story of blindness, but not the *whole* story. They also remind us that insofar as blindness is expressed in the living of a life and expressed throughout the millennia of the evolution and revolution of what, following Arendt (1958), we might call, the 'human condition,' the story of blindness can *never* be told once and for all, and thus cannot be told with the finality of completion. These questions remind us that the story of blindness is told and retold on each and every occasion of experiencing it, of speaking about it, and of thinking about it, and told and retold within the web of the conversation called the human condition.

Coming to understand that the story of blindness is not over in one telling is already the beginning of the development of a mature relation to it. We aim not to be through with blindness until it is through with us, and since it will never be through with us, we must seek to never be through with it. I will be blind for the rest of my life, and blindness will never be through with me. Blindness is present in human existence as a whole, and thus blindness will never be through with humanity.

I have already begun, in the last chapter, to retell the story of passing. This 'retelling' has allowed us to 'see' how blind persons pass without any desire for deception. It is possible for blind persons to pass and *not* deceive others, or themselves, into interpreting them as sighted. Passing becomes more than clinging to a 'sighted' sense of self through the rejection of blindness as a form of self-identity. Let us now continue with the story of passing and continue to treat blindness as a teacher.

Passing in public places is interesting, not because it is done in public, since all passing is, but because it is passing which orients to public places as settings where anyone is visually available to everyone else. People in a public place are constituent features of that place. Each public place has its physical features, such as buildings, sidewalks, and the like, but what makes a place public is the aggregation of people. I am speaking here of places such as city streets, shopping malls, and the like, where people aggregate and do not necessarily know each other or do not necessarily come to that place for any particular oriented group activity.

Passing in places such as these has an orientation which is quite different from passing in a place such as a university department. People in public places are seen by one another but are not necessarily noticed. This is the unique feature of passing in a public place. Being in a public place means being seen but not noticed, and it is *this* that marks the particular challenge for blind persons.

Recall that at one point in my life I had enough residual vision to 'get around' without the use of a white cane or dog guide. At that time, crossing city streets had its unique trouble. I could not see the traffic-lights and thus could not tell, at least from that signal alone, whether or not it was safe for me to cross. I made use of other signals to do so. Traffic flow was one method I used. I listened to and watched the traffic, and, in time, I was able to determine a pattern that indicated whether or not the traffic-light was in my favour. I also attended to pedestrian traffic. Such attention would enable me to see an order in a particular intersection. Whereas people who see watch only the traffic-lights to determine this order, or so I assumed, I attended to the *entire* order of the intersection. It was to this order that I reacted for street crossing and not to the order of traffic-lights. Acting with the assumption that both vehicle and pedestrian traffic would follow such an order, I then crossed the street.

For the most part, this method worked. It relied, however, on a steady traffic flow, and, when this was not present, crossing the street became more difficult. In this situation, other procedures were required. More time was required. I needed to stand on the street corner for a longer time in order to determine the traffic pattern. Even though 'more time' worked as a method for crossing the street, it presented a new difficulty. I may have had to stand at the street corner for quite some time before determining traffic flows, and thus I may have been standing there even though the traffic-light was in my favour. In these instances of passing, I oriented to a public place as a place where I *could* be observed. Standing at a street corner when the traffic-light was in my favour meant that it was possible for me to be noticed as standing there 'for no good reason.' I would be both seen and noticed insofar as standing at the corner for no good reason is noteworthy.

I needed to be seen as standing there 'for a good reason,' thereby diminishing my chances of being noticed. I needed to make my standing on the corner to be seen by others as reasonable. To this end, I often interactionally accomplished 'daydreaming.' I would look up or in some other direction in a wistful way. When I determined that it was safe for me to cross the street, I would then 'snap out' of my daydream and cross. I would be seen in a way that anyone else would be seen if they were day-dreaming at a street crossing only to suddenly realize that they could cross.

Another method I employed, which incidentally I preferred, was the procedure of 'waiting.' I leaned against an object near the street corner, such as a post or newspaper stand. I then acted as if I were waiting for someone while, all the time, attending to the traffic flow. Once I deter-mined that it was safe for me to cross, I acted as if I had become impatient with waiting by looking impatiently at my wrist-watch, and, having decided not to wait any longer, crossed the street.

Activities such as daydreaming or waiting are activities that people sometimes do in public places. These activities are often seen but not nec-essarily noticed, at least not noticed as puzzling or, in some other way, troubling. They are merely activities, among a myriad of others, that are engaged in by people in public places.

I did a similar sort of interactional work when I confronted a set of stairs in a public place. Although my residual vision allowed me, more often than not, to see that I was approaching a set of stairs, it did not allow me to see *precisely* where the stairs began. This situation presented me with difficulty, particularly with a set of stairs leading downwards. A feature of a public place is that people are able to manipulate stairways, doors, etc., without being noticed. Like many other activities in the world, manoeuvring down stairs and through doors are activities which are taken for granted and thus are unproblematic. These are ordinary activi-ties engaged in by ordinary people. For most, the problematic character of manoeuvring up or down a stairway would never be noticed were it not for extraordinary features such as wheelchair ramps.

Deciding to pass meant that I needed to manoeuvre stairways in such a way that made it appear as if the manoeuvre was unproblematic. I could not see where, in a precise way, the stairs began. In order not to fall down the stairs and to manipulate them in an interactionally unproblematic way, I had to locate the point at which the stairs began. Much like the situation of crossing streets, I did what people often do in public places – I 'reminded' myself of something. I approached the stairs to their approximate starting point. I then 'snapped my fingers' and reminded myself of something while, all along, feeling for the first stair with my foot. Having reminded myself of something and having located where the stairs began, I then proceeded down them.

I often used another method for proceeding down stairs, a method which, however, required a prop. I needed to be carrying something such as a bag, a briefcase, or the like. This method was similar to the method of 'reminding.' When I approached the stairs, I stopped and looked in my bag or briefcase to make sure that I had the article that I needed. I searched for the first stair with my foot while 'looking' for the article. Having found the article, which, of course, coincided with finding the first stair, I then proceeded down.

What do these instances of passing teach us? Do we learn only that blind people with residual vision pass as sighted in public places? Do we learn that a form of passing is engaged in even by those who are totally blind when they look toward the voice of someone with whom they are speaking? We do learn this. But we learn more.

We learn that everyone, blind or sighted, orients to public places in a similar way. All of us orient to public places as places in which we are seen but unnoticed. People sometimes stumble, apparently on nothing, when they walk down a sidewalk. Rather than being 'noticed' as someone who is clumsy, we often look at our shoe or back at the place we stumbled as a way to publicly demonstrate that we stumbled 'for a good reason.' We typically understand ourselves, while in public places, as *features* of those places. All of us know that we are *particular* people in a public place. Some of us are clumsy, some graceful, some sighted, and still others blind. Despite our particularity, we typically desire to keep our particularity to ourselves while in a public place and thus be seen only as features of such places.

Thus, all of us pass in public places. Unless we want to be noticed, we keep our particularity to ourselves by passing as 'just one more person' in the aggregate of people in a public place. This is what makes 'people watching' an interesting activity for some. What is being 'watched for' is the unique particularity of a person in a public place that typically goes unnoticed.

This version of passing is not animated by deception. No one, whether sighted or not, passes in a public place as a method for deceiving others into thinking that he or she has no uniqueness or no particularity. While in a public place, we assume that everyone has a particularity, and we assume that everyone desires to keep that particularity to themselves. Announcing something particular while in a public place would itself be noticed as 'odd.' It would be odd if someone, while walking on a busy city sidewalk, stopped everyone and announced that she or he was married. It would be difficult, if not impossible, for the person doing so to account for such an action, but he or she would have to give a 'reason' or be interpreted as 'odd.'

We now learn something about the world which the adolescent relation to blindness did not teach. The adolescent relation to blindness, whether in the form of an individual adolescent passing or in the form of the discipline of rehabilitation, conceived the world as 'sighted.' As such, both passing and rehabilitation techniques are animated by a sense of 'fitting in.' Some blind persons fit in by passing as if they can see, while rehabilitation conceives of its techniques of daily living as a way to fit in. Both conceive the world as sighted, and this conception provides no other possibility for blind persons than fitting in.

All of us see the need for fitting in at one time or another. From time to time, we find ourselves in situations of which we are not a part. People who live in a rural area, for example, may visit a city or vice versa. We often try to fit in to city life or rural life. Despite our attempts to fit in and our preferences, we do not conceive the world as *only* city or as *only* rural. We may conceive of ourselves as 'city types' or as 'rural types,' but we do not conceive the world as *either and only* one or the other. We see the world as just that, the world, and see it as encompassing both city and rural settings.

What does passing without deception teach us about the world? We saw from our examples of passing in public places that all of us, blind or sighted, have a unique particularity and that in order to be seen as features of a public place and hence not noticed, we keep our particularity to ourselves.[2] But this is not an example of deception; we are not deceiv-

---

2 Despite this, uniqueness and particularity are often features of public places and are often noticeable. Blindness is noticeable insofar as white canes and dog guides are. These are signs of blindness or, better, 'public signs,' and thus blindness is oriented to in

ing others into thinking that we have no uniqueness. We do not see others in public places as others without particularity. We orient to our home life in a similar, albeit converse, way. We want to be *both* seen and noticed while at home. We are constituent features of our homes, but we are so in terms of our particularity. We expect that those who live with us will orient to us in the particular ways that living intimately expects and not in the anonymous ways of the public place. But we are both; we are the intimate particular persons of home and the relatively anonymous persons of a public place. Still, this does not lead us to conceive the world as *either* a private place *or* a public place. The world remains the world, inhabited with private and public places.

When I passed in a public place, I was not doing so in order to deceive others into thinking I could see. I was doing what people do in public places; I was keeping my particularity, including my blindness, to myself. I was fitting in, like everyone else. I was attempting to cross streets, walk down stairs, and the like, in a way that made these activities seem to be what they essentially were, namely, unproblematic. I treated passing as a method for 'moving through the world' and not as a method for deceiving others into thinking I could see. Passing became a method for being-in-the-world.

The lesson to be learned from this type of passing is buried in the plurality of technique. But we can at least glimpse the lesson. Passing teaches

public. What becomes noticeable in public places is the particularity of the conceptions of blindness. I have been using a dog guide, Smokie, for the past three years. This means that my blindness is noticeable in public. But it also means that conceptions of blindness are now noticeable to me. Since Smokie, the interaction I have in public has increased dramatically. Most of this interaction is directed to Smokie. Thus particular conceptions of blindness become visible. I am often asked if I need help. Many people ask me whether I know where I am or where I am going. A woman on a subway touched me and asked, 'Do you know where you are?' Questions such as these raise particular conceptions of blindness. First, there is the conception that blind persons need help and, second, that we have difficulty orienting to our environment. These questions raise the idea of a 'type.' To what type of person would these questions be put? Who am I? at the moment I am asked such questions? I give one further example. I was looking for a particular cafe, and, recognizing that I was close to it, I asked someone where precisely it was. He told me that it was just a couple of doors down, but that it was a very expensive place. He then informed me that there was a cheap doughnut shop nearby and disappeared. These are just some examples of particularity *vis-à-vis* blindness that are noticeable in public. Thus, blind persons are *not* noticed without collective representations. When we notice a blind person, we notice ourselves insofar as our conceptions of blindness provide for each noticing of blind persons.

us that the conception 'sighted world' is a metaphor. It metaphorically points to sight as the natural order of things. It points to the quantitative understanding that most people see. It metaphorically represents the need for blind persons to fit into the realm of public experience. This means that it metaphorically points to the recommendation that private experience must be lived and unfolded as part of the realm of public life. Passing teaches us that the world is *neither* sighted *nor* blind. It teaches us that the world *is* the world because it is constituted within the multiplicity of gender, race, disability, and the like. The world has men and women in it, blind persons and sighted persons in it, and so on.

Metaphors such as 'sighted world' and 'male world' are thus not descriptive in the way adolescence would have it. Instead, these metaphors make reference to versions of influence, hegemony, power, and exploitation. The world is composed of points of view and opinion. It is when one opinion, or one point of view, presents itself as 'descriptive fidelity' that metaphors such as these come into play. Passing teaches us that describing the world as 'sighted,' or as 'male,' *must* be hegemonic since the world is neither of these things. The descriptor 'sighted world' is a gloss for the disablist point of view which holds out nothing other for blind persons than fitting in. The point of view of sexism also makes use of the descriptor 'male world' as a way to hold out no other option for women than to fit in. Both descriptors recommend a particular way of fitting in – a way that reconfirms and maintains the world as sighted and as male.

The use of the descriptor 'sighted world' is not restricted to persons who see. The 'sighted world' is not a point of view that derives only from the viewpoint of sightedness. When blindness is conceived as no view at all or conceived as no point from which to view, only one point of view remains – sightedness. This is the point of view of the adolescent relation to blindness. This is the view seen from the viewpoint of the blind person who passes 'as if' she or he can see. This is also the view seen from the viewpoint of the blind person who understands him- or herself as not passing. This is the view seen by those blind persons who 'look' toward the voice and thus make 'eye contact' with those to whom they are speaking, while all along displaying a white cane, and who 'see' this method *only* as a method for fitting into the world and not as a method for demonstrating their essential *place* in it.

Passing teaches us that blindness belongs in, and to, the world. It teaches us that, in the midst of all the points of view to the contrary, blindness has a place in the world and that its requirement is the making and remaking of that place. Unlike fitting in, which requires the flexibility of adaptation, making a place requires *imagining* that place. It requires imagining a life as blind rather than merely adapting to that life. Let me illustrate this by quoting Cicero (1971, 110–11):

Take blindness. What pleasures, in fact, does this dreaded condition deprive you of? Whereas all the other pleasures are actually located in the organs of sensation, it has been pointed out that the contrary applies to visual perception, which does not cause any direct pleasure to the eyes themselves in the same way as taste, smell, touch and hearing gratify the appropriate organs in which each of those senses is localized. In the case of the eyes, however, the situation is different, because our visual impressions are not destined for them at all, but for the mind.

And the mind is capable of receiving a wide and varied range of satisfaction in which sight is not involved in any way whatever. I am speaking of education, culti-vated people, the sort of person for whom life means thought: and a wise man rarely needs the support of his eyes in order to think. Happiness does not come to an end at the conclusion of every day, when night falls; so why should it cease when blindness turns day into night? On this subject Antipater the Cyrenaic made an apt remark, though it is admittedly a trifle coarse. When he heard his women folk moaning because he was blind, his answer was this: 'What's the matter? Don't you think one can have a good time in the night?'

Cicero speaks of blindness by initially addressing the conventional con-ception of it as lack. (Remember that Cicero wrote these lines over two thousand years ago, and what is interesting about this is that this same conception of blindness pervades our individual and collective conscious-ness even today, meaning that such a conception cannot be shaken even over the passage of two millennia.) The complaint that the conception of lack levels against blindness is that it deprives the one who is blind. It is toward this complaint that Cicero aims his remarks.

Cicero hears the complaint against blindness as centring on pleasure; blindness deprives one of pleasure. However, he cannot imagine how blindness can deprive anyone of pleasure. There is no pleasure to be felt in the eye when it sees, and blindness alone[3] certainly does not deprive anyone of the pleasures of education, cultivation, or thought. Cicero says that blindness deprives neither the body nor the mind of its particular pleasures.

The destiny of visual perception is the mind, is thought. Even though

---

3 Blind persons have been deprived of education *but* deprived of this by others, most often others who see.

visual perception is destined for thought, vision itself is not a necessary condition for thought. It is implied in Cicero's thoughts about blindness that visual perception is not 'pre-destined' for thought; visual perception may or may not fulfil its destiny. Destined as it is for thought, visual perception, or the lack of it, neither determines thought nor deprives one of the need for a thoughtful life. As Cicero says, '... a wise man rarely needs the support of his eyes in order to think.'

Eyes are not the source of thought; they neither engender thought nor support the need to think. If what the eyes see is destined for the mind, then perception must be what the eyes make out of what they see. Presumably, the brain already does, at least, a version of this by neurologically producing visual images, and does this without any attention from the mind. Our brains produce visual images in much the same way that our bodies produce breathing. No thought, at least in the way Cicero was speaking of it, is required either for the production of visual images or breathing. When Cicero says that visual perceptions are destined for the mind, he must be speaking about some need to make something of these perceptions or to think about what we are seeing. And, to think about the images given to us by our eyes certainly does not require their support.

If Cicero was right when he said that a wise person rarely needs the support of eyes to think, then it follows that a person who was 'not wise' would, first, not be inclined to think, not be inclined to the thoughtful life; and, second, *would* require the support of eyes for the life without thought. The unthoughtful life would be *satisfied* with the visual images it sees. The life without thought would be satisfied with a 'sensual finality' – a finality that ends, and ironically begins, with the sheer sensual experience of the world. Living unthoughtfully means living a life in, what Kierkegaard calls, the sheer 'immediacy' of life. The 'immediate person' almost always requires the support of eyes to live in-immediacy.

Without the support of eyes, this sensual finality and immediacy would be difficult, if not impossible. This is the sort of lack or deprivation which grounds the complaint against blindness. This is the 'truth' that lies behind the lamentation of blindness – the truth which celebrates the satisfaction of sensual finality and immediacy. Without the support of eyes, this life is impossible.

This is the lament of Antipater's 'women folk.' They bemoaned the fact that, because of his blindness, Antipater could no longer live with sensual finality and could no longer live in-immediacy. His 'women folk' bemoaned Antipater's blindness since they could not imagine a blind person having a 'good time.' For them, 'a good time is had by all' if, and *only* if, *all can see*. But in the face of blindness, Antipater's womenfolk can only moan. The only way they can imagine responding to blindness is with pity. Antipater is pitied because he is blind, and, because he is blind, he deserves the pity that *anyone* who lives without sensual finality deserves. Antipater can no longer experience the satisfaction of the always anticipated, yet unrevealed, surprises of sensuality, and he no longer lives in the sensuality of the 'mystery of the eye.' Given this, who would not pity Antipater?

But in the midst of all of this moaning, Antipater asks, 'What's the matter? Don't you think one can have a good time in the night?' Coarse as it is, this question is Antipater's response to the moaning. Assuming that this moaning represents the response of pity toward blindness, Antipater's question would then be directed toward this response. It would be directed toward pity.

The first thing we notice about Antipater's response is that it is offered in the form of a question. He could have responded in other ways. He could have responded by joining with his womenfolk and bemoaned his own blindness. He could have responded to pity with pity by commiserating with it through self-pity. Or he could have responded with anger and berated his womenfolk for feeling sorry for him. And we could imagine many other responses. The point is that in the midst of a myriad of possible responses, he *chose* a question.

What is Antipater asking or saying with his question? His question can be heard as asking for the women's opinion regarding the relation between blindness and a good time. But his question seems more rhetorical than this. Antipater's question seems to spring more from a motive to tell the women something than to ask them something. Antipater's question raises the relation between blindness and a good time, a relation of which the moaning makes use but does not raise. This is one of the pitiful things about pity. It typically assumes and presupposes the need for pity without raising, or questioning, this need. Pity does not often raise the decisive character of itself and does not examine its *own* conception of blindness, a conception which makes the response of pity possible in the first place. Pity understands itself as a response *to some thing*. It sees this *thing* as something external to it and as something objective insofar as pity conceives of it without considering this 'conceiving.' Pity thinks of blindness, without thinking it is thinking, as something to be pitied and as something that *anyone,* including blind persons themselves, would pity. Pity never considers blindness in terms of 'possibilities,' and this is what makes pity so pitiful.

Antipater's question, more than merely asking for the opinion of the womenfolk, questions pity itself. Rather than asking for their opinion, an opinion Antipater already received through their moaning, he questions it. Antipater already knows why his womenfolk are moaning. He already knows why they feel sorry for him. They pity him because he is blind. They see nothing good about being blind and thus have nothing but pity for those who are. Antipater knows this and knows, too, that *this* could be otherwise. He also knows that the womenfolk do not know this.

Antipater raises a conception of blindness which is *opposite* to that held by pity. His question raises the possibility of having a good time in the night, of having a good time *in blindness*. In the same way Cicero himself did, Antipater raises this possibility by invoking the analogy of day and night. In chapter 4, Parisian raised an alternative conception of blindness by demonstrating how he could 'do things' and that the 'doing of these things' displayed to others as well as to himself his competence. Parisian's response to pity was competence. In contrast, Antipater's response is that of 'good times,' joy, happiness. Parisian's question to pity would be quite different from that of Antipater, although equally as coarse, since Parisian would ask, 'What's the matter? Don't you think one can be competent in the night?'

Competence does not necessarily bring joy or happiness. There are many things we do competently without necessarily enjoying them. It is, however, difficult to imagine having a good time without enjoying it. Doing things, and having a good time doing them, brings with it a sense of enjoyment, while doing things competently brings with it a sense of accomplishment but not necessarily joy. Doing things competently while, at the same time, enjoying them brings both a sense of accomplishment and joy.

Antipater's question raises the possibility not only of having a good time in the night but also of enjoying the life of blindness, enjoying being 'in the night.' This possibility is something which pity cannot imagine. *And this is precisely what Antipater's question seeks to tell pity.* This question tells pity that it cannot imagine blindness, first of all, as a life and, second, as a life that can be lived with joy and happiness. Even though pity cannot imagine this, it can imagine the opposite; hence, moaning. Thus Antipater's question seeks to remind pity of what it does and does not imagine.

In responding to pity, Antipater invokes an analogy. He did not respond with anger nor did he chide his womenfolk for feeling sorry for him, and he did not respond to their pity with assurance by saying something like 'Don't worry. I'll be all right.' Not only were these responses available to Antipater as alternatives to his question, but they are also responses that many blind people use in the face of pity. A blind woman, Anne, told me of an incident she experienced at a Las Vegas casino:

I was just standing there. I had my white cane and I was just waiting for my friend. I don't know, maybe I looked a little odd because I was quite excited. You know, I just won $2,400 and I had it in my purse. I don't even think I realized it at the time but I was also holding that little cup, you know, that thing they give you for coins. If you can believe this, someone walked by and put some money in that cup. I said, 'No, no, it's okay.' But the guy insisted. He said it was tough enough being sighted in this city and it must be even tougher being blind. I told him I was okay, but then he was gone. There I was with $2,400 in my purse and the guy's putting some money in my cup. You never get away from that, people just think that if you're blind they have to feel sorry for you.

Ignoring the sheer irony of this story, if that is possible, we notice that Anne, unlike Antipater, chose to respond to pity with assurance. Anne tried to assure the 'guy' that she was 'okay' and did not need his money. Despite her protestations and her attempt to assure him, he insisted that Anne needed pity and, having given her some, went on his way. Like Antipater's womenfolk, this 'guy' could not imagine having a good time in Las Vegas 'in the night.' The irony of this situation is that Anne had just won over two thousand dollars, and this is certainly one indicator of having had a 'good time' in Las Vegas and having it in the night. The 'guy' did not consider what having a good time in Las Vegas would mean 'in the night' or, for that matter, 'in the day.' His pity could not imagine anyone having a good time in the night, *in blindness*. He heard Anne's response as an attempt to assure him that despite the fact that she was not having a good time in the night, she was 'okay.' Anne's response was open to the interpretation that, despite living in the night, blind persons can, and do, adapt.

In contrast, Antipater's question was an attempt to *tell* pity of the necessity to *imagine* a *life in blindness*. The question of adaptation was put to one side since blind persons adapt and find ways to do things and to do them well. But to enjoy doing things and to have a good time is another question, a question that Antipater raises. This question raises the need for imagination insofar as it is necessary to imagine a life *in blindness* that goes beyond the development of competence. It raises the question not only of imagining a 'good time' but, as Cicero says, imagining the life of 'cultivation' and of 'thought.' Antipater's question reminds us of the need to imagine a thoughtful and enjoyable relation to the life *in blindness*.

What represents a mature relation to blindness is that Antipater's question is a reminder to himself. He reminds himself of the temptation of pity in relation to his blindness. Cicero was right when he said that happiness does not end with the conclusion of the day. But the day does succumb to nightfall, and the night to daybreak. Even the insomniac knows that the darkness of night will be broken by the light of day. One follows the other and rarely does one come and stay. The insomniac knows, and knows only too well, the terror of the 'never-ending day.'[4] The never-ending night poses a similar terror to blind persons. This is the temptation that pity holds out to blindness. It tempts blindness to see itself as the quintessential terror of the insomniac, namely, to see itself as a never-ending night. As such, blindness *should* be bemoaned. Hence the need for Antipater's question.

Antipater's question also alludes to competence in relation to blindness. There is no question that, when blind, some of the things we enjoy doing may be difficult, and some, even impossible. But many blind persons find ways to do the things they enjoy. There are many ways to read, and the 'sound' of words, as they resonate in a person's voice, are sometimes even more enjoyable than their 'visual appearance.' Still, reading is a visual event steeped in the sensuality of the 'look' of reading materials, in particular, the look of print, its organization, its size, its design, and the rest, and it is also the look of a book jacket, of its cover design, of its size and shape, and the like. Together with this 'look' comes the tactile sense of reading materials, the feel of the book, the turning of pages, the almost oblivious reaching for some other object, such as a beverage, the reaching for a book on a desk or bookshelf, and all the rest of the tactile sensuality of reading. The eyes, as Cicero said, feel none of this but see it all. And all of this is destined for the mind.

A blind person reads, but reads only when the visual event of reading is transformed into an 'aural event.'[5] The process of this transformation removes the visual sense of reading and, to a lesser extent, the tactile sense. If the senses of vision and touch are an essential part of reading, and an essential part of its enjoyment, then the enjoyment of reading is affected by the diminishing of these sensations. The enjoyableness of reading, when blind, is transformed much in the way that the visual event

---

4 For an excellent analysis of the relation between insomnia and postmodernism, see McHugh 1994.

5 I have examined this phenomenon in detail in my 'Reading Aloud' (1978). This analysis, of course, would be different if Braille was used as the example.

of reading is transformed into an aural event insofar as reading silently to oneself is transformed into a listening. This reading, too, has its sensuality but not that of vision or, to a lesser degree, that of touch (this is why some blind persons prefer Braille). The sensuality connected to reading aloud comes from the sense of hearing – hearing a book being read aloud, thus hearing words, sentences, and paragraphs, and even punctuation and italics, and hearing what the author 'says' as a transformation of what the author 'wrote.' For the blind person, there is a more direct relation to the 'challenge' of reading, a challenge which marks the enjoyment of reading, namely, the challenge of *hearing* what the author is *saying*.

Competence in relation to reading assumes, but is superseded by, the desire to hear what the author is saying. The enjoyableness of reading stems from a thoughtful rather than from a mechanical reading. A 'wise reader' rarely needs the support of eyes to read thoughtfully. This is why the issue of accessibility must not be the goal or end of a relation to blindness. Having *access* to books is one thing; reading them thoughtfully is another. The issue of accessibility takes on a different meaning. Typically, accessibility is thought of by conceiving the world as sighted and by addressing the technical problem of making that world accessible to blind persons. The goal or end of such a conception of accessibility is the living of an ordinary life. Other than living it, however, what do we make of this ordinary life? The question for a blind person becomes Now that I have access to ordinary life and can live it more or less ordinarily, what do I make of it and how do I enjoy it? Both blind and sighted persons can ask, What do blind persons 'see' when they 'see' ordinary life?

Let us return once more to Cicero as a way to address this question. Homer is traditionally said to be blind. 'But,' writes Cicero (ibid., 112),

... when we read what he wrote, it seems more than poetry; it is as distinct as if he had painted the whole thing. So vividly, indeed, has he depicted every region and sea-coast and locality in Greece, every shape and form of warfare and battle, every manoeuvre which a ship can possibly make, every possible activity of men or beasts, that he gives us the most brilliantly clear vision of all the things his blindness prevented him from seeing himself. Surely, then, we are not going to suppose that Homer lacked pleasure or enjoyment!

Cicero was impressed with Homer's vivid depictions and with the brilliantly clear vision he gives of the things he himself was prevented from seeing. Even though Homer was prevented from seeing the things he depicted, Cicero did not speak of this in terms of lack. He spoke of

Homer's blindness in terms of 'prevention.' Homer was prevented from seeing things he depicted in the same way that we are prevented by mortality from the possibility of living forever, even though that same mortality provides for the possibility of life in the first place. Mortality need not be conceived as lack. In the same way, Cicero was recommending that blindness need not be conceived as lack.

For Cicero, the prerequisites for a 'vivid depiction' are pleasure and enjoyment. So vivid are his depictions of Homer that Cicero gives us the brilliantly clear vision that such depiction is rarely needful of the support of eyes. Homer's depictions do not lack vision even though he himself was prevented from seeing what he depicted. While not being born of vision, Homer's depictions give birth to a brilliantly clear vision.

In fact, Cicero himself, because of place and time of birth, was also prevented from seeing what Homer depicted. But, this does not mean that Cicero lacked pleasure or enjoyment. His depiction of Homer resonates with as much pleasure and enjoyment as does Homer's depiction of Greece. Cicero's enjoyment of Homer's work can be located in the pleasure he finds with Homer's engagement with depiction, *depict(us)*, with his vivid 'word painting' of Greece. Cicero enjoys the irony of Homer's depiction, and he (Cicero) himself finds pleasure and enjoyment through depicting the irony of a blind person creating a brilliantly clear vision. Cicero makes use of Homer's depiction of Greece to depict blindness as the joy of living ironically in the world. He is not so much impressed with Homer's competence in describing the sights of Greece, the manoeuvres of ships, battles, etc., as he is with Homer's ironic relation to that which he depicts. Cicero is saying that it is only such a relation (irony) that leads to a vividness of vision which, in turn, 'gives' a brilliantly clear depiction. Thus Homer's 'perception' fulfilled its destiny in the mind, in thought, and this, ironically, even though he was blind. From this, it is clear that Homer and, ironically, Cicero as well have a good time *in blindness*. Homer has a good time depicting Greece, and Cicero has a good time in depicting Homer, even though both are prevented from seeing what they depict. Both recognize the pleasure and enjoyment of depiction, which includes the irony of any depiction as itself a depiction.

When Cicero says that Homer does not lack pleasure or enjoyment, he is not suggesting that blindness itself is either pleasurable or enjoyable. Cicero is not saying that blindness *comes with* pleasure and enjoyment, but he is saying that blindness is not *without* them. Blindness does not prevent 'looking,' even though it prevents 'seeing.' Without seeing, Homer *engages* the world through depicting what he is 'looking at.' Homer knows that sight neither privileges nor supports the capturing of reality since he knows that reality is always-already depiction. He knows this in the way that Socrates knows that he cannot give Glaucon the 'Good' in an empirical sense but can only give it through a simile, a story; he can only depict it (*Republic*, book 7).

Homer's blindness does not prevent him from depicting Greek life and does not prevent him from 'looking at' the Greek life he desires to depict. His perception of Greek life, a perception which Cicero says is destined for the mind, is what Homer remakes in the form of his depiction of that life. Homer's depiction is vivid and presents a brilliantly clear vision of Greek life. But how could it have been otherwise? Homer must have intended his work to be listened to, and it was subsequently read; he must have understood his work as destined for the mind of his listeners and subsequent readers. Destined for the mind and for thought, Homer's depiction of Greek life, like that life itself, had to be vivid and had to provide for the possibility of the mind receiving a brilliantly clear vision of life. Seeing Greek life, or any life for that matter, with the eyes does not necessarily mean seeing the *animus* of that life. The animus of a life can *only* be glimpsed through thought and thus can only be imitated (depicted) in speech. The irony of such depiction is that it itself depicts the understanding that we are able to glimpse the very thing our eyes prevent us from seeing. Perhaps even more ironic than this, Homer teaches us that in order to depict that which we are prevented from seeing, we *need* the support of the eyes.

For Homer, or for any other blind person for that matter, blindness, despite whatever else it might be, is not a foreign language. Variation in perception aside, blindness and sightedness do not speak separate languages foreign to one another. The visual perceptions of each are often translated for each other, but the language remains the same. Recall that in chapter 3 I spoke about how blind persons use phrases such as 'see you later,' and the like. In usages such as these, blindness draws our ear to a literal sense of everyday language use. Blindness does draw our attention to a correspondence interpretation of language in which speaking corresponds to competence. It is as though blindness points out the oddity of saying something without being able to do it. The 'see' in 'see you later' is interpreted literally rather than in its typical situated interpretation as the termination of a conversation between interlocutors. Nonetheless, a correspondence understanding of language is odd. It would be odd for a blind person to invoke competence and say, instead of 'see you later,' 'feel you later' or 'hear you later.' Even though blindness tempts us to hear everyday language use in a literal way, it simultaneously displays the oddity of such a hearing as well as the limits of any correspondence theory of language.

It is such a correspondence understanding of language that permits for an interpretation of Homer, or of the speech of any other blind person, as passing. Both the *Odyssey* and the *Iliad* can be read as Homer speaking about things of which he knows nothing. But Homer speaks vividly about these things and, as Cicero says, gives us a brilliantly clear vision of them.

Reading Homer's work as a 'description' rather than as a 'depiction' of Greek life leads to a questioning of his competence as a describer since 'seeing' what we describe is typically conceived as an essential feature of description. The same sort of questioning would occur if a blind person described an event such as a movie. Descriptions of 'visual events' are *always* seen as flawed in the absence of sight. It is tantamount to describing an experience never having experienced it. Such critical interpretations may be valid if the aim of speech or writing is description. Even so, the activity of describing possesses an implicit grammar which must also be present if describing is to be 'seen' as such. Part of this grammar is the presence of the describer to the experience, event, or situation he or she is describing.

It is precisely this grammar of description that provides for the possibility of reading Homer's work as an instance of passing and thus as some implicit claim, on his part, of having seen the life he describes. There is no doubt that, as a Greek, Homer experienced Greek life. But because his description is so vivid, Homer can be read as speaking as if he had experienced Greek life visually. Read through the eyes of passing, Homer is conceived as one who speaks outside the realm of visual experience and thus is one who copies the experience of others, hence depicting his desire to fit in by doing what others ordinarily do, namely, describe.

But even when read as description, Homer's work represents neither 'ordinary description' nor a description of 'ordinary things.' Cicero certainly remarks on the extraordinariness of Homer's work. But his remarks do not suggest anything remarkable about Homer's ability to fit into Greek life. Instead, Cicero finds Homer's depiction of Greek life remarkable. Homer's work leads Cicero to remark that blindness need not be conceived as deprivation or as lack. Cicero conceives the good life as the wisdom that desires education and cultivation. The good life is the need for a thoughtful life. Blindness does not deprive anyone of the pleasure and enjoyment of the life of thought. This is probably why Cicero reads Homer's work as depiction rather than as description. Depiction always-already involves more, and goes beyond, the mechanics of description, and when description is done, it is always in the service of depiction.

The phenomenon of passing can also be read as depiction. I have been doing so throughout this work albeit in an indirect way. I spoke about passing as a representation of an adolescent desire to fit in when deception animates it. I spoke, too, about passing in a more mature sense, when deception was absent but passing represented the same desire to fit in. I spoke of passing, both in its adolescent and mature sense, as representing not only a desire to fit into the world but also a desire to represent a knowledge of the world conceived as sighted, knowledge one can possess despite being prevented from seeing it. I have been speaking of passing as representing the possibility of knowledge in the face of deprivation and lack.

But what if we understood passing as depiction in a more direct sense than this? What sort of depiction would passing be and what would it depict? Read as depiction, Homer's work depicted both Greek life in particular as well as life in general. Does passing do the same? Does it depict something in particular and something in general?

Passing is certainly a vivid depiction. Passing, whether that spoken of here or elsewhere,[6] vividly depicts a clear understanding of the situation as well as a clear sense of how the situation is interactionally accomplished. It also depicts an incredibly high level of energy on the part of the passer – an energy tightly concentrated by the clear and tight focus of a single-minded aim to represent oneself as a legitimate member of a situation or setting. Vivid, too, is the depiction of the sly-like cleverness evoked by passers to trick others into believing that they are what they interactionally claim to be. Passers act and interact as if they were ... and the cleverness is depicted in the way others treat them as if they were ... Cleverness is most vividly depicted in the way passers trick sight into 'seeing' blindness as an instance of itself.

Perhaps passing's most vivid depiction is of ordinary life. Any blind person who passes for sighted has some sense that sighted persons do the same insofar as they, too, must show each other and themselves that they are sighted. Persons who see must act as if they can see in order to be seen as seeing. Each passing technique used by a blind person derives from those used by sighted persons. The difference is that whereas blind

6 I mean any example of passing found in the notion of the 'imposter.'

persons make explicit use of these techniques, sighted persons do not. It is in this sense that blindness often provides a more vivid depiction of ordinary seeing life than does sightedness. The presence of blindness often serves as a reminder: it reminds sight that it can see and of what it can see. Blindness often makes sight mindful of the appreciation it has for the pleasure of sensual finality. Passing's depiction of ordinary-seeing-life gives us a brilliantly clear vision of how sight recognizes itself as such as well as of its meaning. The passer does this without the support of eyes. But through the figure of passing, blindness immerses itself in the mystery of the eye while lurking in its shadow.

In its more mature expression, blindness brings the mystery of the eye to the fore and begins to unravel it. The mystery of the eye, which is made manifest through all of its mysterious looks, is generated by the eye's essential inability to see itself. The eye cannot look into itself. The only look that the eye has of itself is when it looks into the eyes of others or when it looks into a mirror. The eye can only see its image and thus can only imagine itself. The eye resembles the self insofar as, like the eye, the self can see itself only through imagination. The self lives within the same shroud of mystery as does the eye. The eye alludes its look in the way the self alludes itself.

The mystery of the eye makes reference to the gap between the eye and the eye of an other or between the eye and its image. Turning its look toward itself means that the eye develops an imaginative relation to itself and thus sees itself within the imaginary of what it means to see (Lacan 1977, 1–7). The mystery of the eye resides in the gap between the eye and its look shrouded in the mystery of the imaginary. The eye's mystery is revealed through its looks and through what it looks at when it sees. It shows itself through the shadow of its image, through the shadows cast by the imaginative relation to the 'look of the eye.'

Maturity understands blindness not as a mere shadow of sight. Instead, blindness is yet one more shadow cast by the eye. It reveals the eye shrouded in mystery. Thus, blindness is no more a shadow than is sight-edness. Blindness is not a shadow of sight but is, like sight itself, cast in the mystery of the eye destined for the development of an imaginative relation to perception, to making and remaking something of the world and to making and remaking its place in it. Blindness is destined for the mind, destined to look at the shadows cast by the mystery of the eye, and destined to look at itself in the midst of the shadows which prevent it from seeing. Blindness shares this destiny with sight.

Even in its most mature expression, blindness is yet one more depiction of the mystery of the eye. The uniqueness of blindness is not grounded in its distinctiveness from sight conceived in terms of opposition. What distinguishes it from sight is the revelation of the fundamental anxiety which springs from the understanding that it is prevented from seeing what it depicts. This is the quintessential lesson that blindness, through the figure of passing, teaches. Blindness can teach this to the one *in blindness* as well as to the one *in sightedness*.

Blindness is not opposed to sight in the way sight is opposed to it. Sightedness and blindness are not related to one another through the opposition of one who sees and one who does not. This opposition covers over the more fundamental one against looking at that which cannot be seen. It is the opposition inherent in the Socratic understanding of knowing that we do not know, and the one inherent in 'seeing that we do not see.'

Homer's vivid depiction of Greek life can be read as his attempt to live with this paradox. Homer understands that he cannot 'see' Greek life, not because blindness prevents him from doing so, but because the life of Greece lies behind the multitude of scenes, events, and activities of that life and is thus not an empirical object there for anyone to see. Greek life, therefore, *must* be a formulation. The scenes, events, and activities of that life must be re-formed with the aim of providing a depiction of the particular character of what can then, and *only* then, be called 'Greek life.' We should not be impressed with Homer's depiction because his blindness prevented him from seeing what he depicted since *no Greek*, blind or sighted, has ever been able to see what he or she has depicted. What *is* impressive about Homer's work is its display of commitment to depiction – its commitment to 'bringing into view' that which is impossible to see. Homer's work represents a life committed to inquiry or to, what Socrates called, the 'examined life' (Plato, *Apology*). It is a life that displays the ironic tension of always straining to see that which cannot be in focus. Homer's blindness depicts the travail of such a maieutic enterprise by testing and trying his commitment to it.

Passing in its most mature expression recommends a relation to blindness that is committed to living with the paradox of seeing that it cannot see. The life of sightedness and the life of blindness are not empirical objects and thus cannot be seen. If they are objects at all, they are objects of thought, and, as Cicero said, thought rarely needs the support of the eyes. But, depiction is another story. It is the bringing of invisible thought into view. If Plato is right and thought is the imitation of the movement in the soul (*Theaetetus*), then depiction is the imitation of thought. As an embodiment of thought, speech requires the body and, as such, requires sensory metaphor whether or not the senses are concretely present in the speaker. This is why Homer's work, his speech, needed the support of the eyes.

Karatheodoris's question What is blindness? *must* be read as a provocative invitation. His question invites us to examine our relations to blindness, whether these relations are expressed in regards to the blindness of others or to our own. Karatheodoris provokes us to bring into view our conceptions of blindness, which are imitated in our actions and interactions. He raises the question of blindness in a way similar to Cicero. Karatheodoris suggests that our relations with blindness are destined for the mind insofar as they implicitly provide an answer to the question What is blindness? Our discovery, diagnosis, and subsequent treatment of blindness are themselves destined for the mind in that they all embody particular social relations to blindness and thus provide some answer to the question of blindness as raised by Karatheodoris. His question recommends that blindness is *always a question*. Every relation to, and every action and interaction with, blindness represents an answer to the question of blindness, and every such answer, in turn, since it too represents a relation to blindness, asks once again, and for the first time, What is blindness?[7]

Karatheodoris's question provokes us to see blindness as an open question expressed in the never-ending dialogue between question and answer. His question provokes us to develop the mature relation to blindness which recommends that we live within the ironic paradox of knowing that we do not know blindness and seeing that we do not see it. We must allow blindness to be continuously open to the influence of collective representations and to the multiplicity of opinion in regard to it. We must orient to this multiplicity as representing various relations to blindness and, as such, various voices in the story of blindness. We must understand our own particular relation to blindness as itself a voice in this dialogue, and we must understand our voice as one which both speaks and listens in the midst of the story of blindness and thus as a voice committed to the on-going development of an imaginative relation to what it means to be blind. Finally, and this is the heart of the matter, we must understand our own blindness – the way we conceive it and the way we

---

7 Derrida (1978, 47) speaks of an answer to a question as itself a question. He says, 'Before answering this question, or rather before continuing to ask it ...' Thus all answers to the question of blindness keep the question alive.

live it – as a depiction of blindness and as a depiction of the search for the place of blindness in the world.

Blindness and passing take on a mature dimension when we choose to live decisively, that is, to live as if we know and see blindness. We pass as sighted, acting as if we know what blindness is and see its place. Still, we know that we do not know and we see that we do not see, and we pass in order to depict our commitment to the ironically paradoxical life of speakers and actors in the continuously unfolding story of blindness.

Deciding to be such a speaker rarely requires the support of the eyes, but the depiction of such a decision always does. Depiction is not only an activity destined for the mind; it is also an activity *of* the mind. The aim of depiction is to bring that which is invisible into view. Depiction aims at making the invisible visible.[8] Through his depiction, Homer gives a brilliantly clear vision of Greek life, a life which is essentially invisible.

Blindness is also essentially invisible. Even though we see signs of it, such as persons using white canes, using dog guides, reading Braille, etc., we do not see blindness itself. Ophthalmologists see neurological pathology – causes of blindness – but they do not see blindness. Sight is no more able to see blindness than it is able to see itself. Even blind persons cannot see blindness; we experience it through our feelings, through how we are treated by others, through the different ways we have of doing things, and so on, *but we do not see it.*

Even seeing that we do not see blindness does not come from sense perception. Eyes do not allow for such a vision. We see this only through thought. Bringing this thought into view requires depiction, requires the imitation of thought through speech and action. This is why whatever is said about blindness, be it said by ophthalmology, rehabilitation, or by blind persons, *must* be heard as a depiction. Depictions of blindness can be judged for their vividness, their clarity, and their need to speak of blindness without being the final word. This understanding allows for blind persons to conceive their speech and action as depictions of the life of blindness. We have seen such depictions throughout this work: we have seen how adolescence depicts blindness as making reference to the desire for collective life; how ophthalmology depicts it as a 'hopeless case' requiring human adaptation; and we have seen how rehabilitation depicts blindness as a nuisance to be manoeuvred around on the road of participation in the sighted world.

All of these depictions give a vision of blindness as nuisance, and,

8 See Arendt 1971, especially pages 19–128.

indeed, we can often see this vision clearly. Blindness is a nuisance in the desire to sense the world visually. It is certainly a nuisance to a normally functioning physiology. Blindness is a nuisance to any desire for adolescent collective life, and it is undoubtedly a nuisance which stands in the way of the desire to do the ordinary things of ordinary life.

Despite the clarity of this vision, 'nuisance' depicts blindness as deprivation and lack. What blindness deprives one of is a 'clear road' on which one can ordinarily travel and travel unencumbered. Blindness deprives one of the taken-for-granted clarity that comes with ordinary sense perception, the doing of ordinary things, and the experiencing of ordinary experiences.

However, a mature relation to blindness understands that, however blindness is lived, the life of blindness *is* a depiction. Blindness is a reflexive phenomenon insofar as the *living* of blindness reflects a conception of what it is. This is what the mature passer sees and understands. The mature passer speaks and acts decisively *vis-à-vis* blindness insofar as he or she lives as if he or she sees and knows blindness. This is why the mature passer can sometimes act as if he or she were sighted and, at other times, not.

Living decisively with blindness is represented by a commitment to depict blindness through conceiving life as a narration of the story of blindness. It is a commitment to telling the story of blindness through the living of a life, even though blindness itself cannot be seen. It is a commitment to passing, to acting as if blindness can be seen while, at the same time, seeing that it cannot. This is the same commitment that Socrates had to, what he called, the Good. He told the story of the Good, thus acting as if he knew the Good, while knowing that he did not.

This is what is meant by a commitment to living the 'examined life.' It is living blindness with the understanding that life is responsible for the appearance of blindness. It appears *only* through our actions and interactions. It appears in our life with blindness and thus appears in the depiction represented in the answer to the question What is blindness? In whatever way blindness appears, we have a hand in making it do so. Those of us who are blind, and who relate to our blindness in a mature way, know that the appearance of blindness is a story and that we are responsible for its telling.

The lesson that blindness can teach sight is that it, too, is a narrative. Blindness can teach sighted persons that they are prevented from seeing sightedness and that their lives, ordinary or not, are depictions of sight represented in the answer to the question What is sight? Blindness can teach sightedness that it, too, passes. Even though sight often thinks it can see everything, it cannot see itself. The lesson is that, like blind persons, sighted persons also pass and act as if they can see. Maturity makes reference to the commitment of living, what Socrates called, the 'examined life' and to, what Cicero called, the 'thoughtful life.' It means thinking about blindness, living it thoughtfully, and responsibly. It means knowing that blindness appears in the world and knowing that this appearance points to blindness but is itself not blindness. It is a commitment to, what the ancient Greeks called, *theoria*, the wonder that mysteriously manifests itself in the shadows of appearances – the wonder of blindness that appears in the world of those who see and of those who do not.

I have tried to speak of a mature relation to blindness and have done so throughout this book. I have tried to represent blindness as a life which narrates a story. The various views of blindness I have given voice to represent different speakers in the story of blindness. I have attempted to bring these voices together under the auspices that blindness is a story. My conception of blindness as a story allowed me, on the one hand, to hear the various voices in the telling of this story and, on the other, to tell the story.

Concluding my story with the idea of a mature relation to blindness does not mean that the other voices in this story have now been silenced. Nothing can be further from the truth. All of these voices, and undoubtedly many more, remain forever in the story of blindness. My infancy, childhood, and adolescence are not over merely because I have already lived through them. Instead, living through them means that they are with me forever. My discovery of blindness, the diagnosis of my blindness, my adolescent blindness, and the rehabilitation of my blindness are with me forever and are voices that I continuously hear. Allowing these voices to speak to me is what generated the writing of this book.

Since I initially discovered my blindness, I have rediscovered it in many ways. My blindness has been diagnosed several times by many ophthalmologists, and, if diagnosis means an evaluation, *my life* as a blind person has been diagnosed many times and by many people, some of whom are blind and some who are not. I am continuously searching for new techniques for doing things, some of which are ordinary and some not so ordinary. Finally, and perhaps most importantly, I continue to experience my blindness in many ways, in ways that may be described as childish at times, adolescent at other times, and even, on some rare occasions, as mature. But what my blindness comes to, now that I have come to it, is the wonder of its mystery, a mystery which is so revealing that it grows more mysterious the more I unravel it.

7

Conclusion

In the words of Hannah Arendt (1968, 104), 'the story reveals the meaning of what otherwise would remain an unbearable sequence of sheer happenings.' Bereft of stories, the human condition would be unbearable. It would be to live *through* the unbearable waiting for the next happening, while living *with* the most current one. Meaning is dropped in favour of bearing a current condition while waiting unbearably and preparing for the next.

This is what usually happens to blindness; its meaning is shoved to the side in order to make room for accepting it and adjusting to it. It becomes merely one happening in the sheer sequence of happenstance. The only thing left to do is to make blindness one of those happenings which is relatively easy to bear. It is to make it an ordinary nuisance.

Rather than adopting this view of the human condition and of blindness, I have attempted to address it. I tried to tell the story of blindness and thus to reveal its meaning. My abiding commitment was to elevate blindness from the quagmire of sheer happenstance into the endless horizon of meaning. The story I tell in this book is the story of blindness as it was revealed to me.

It is only fitting that I conclude with a story. Ordinariness has been a significant voice throughout my narration. This voice tells a fascinating story, but only if we do not hear it as the sheer happenstance of the commonplace. Arendt says,

The common and the ordinary must remain our primary concern, the daily food of our thought – if only because it is from them that the uncommon and the extraordinary emerge, and not from matters that are difficult and sophisticated. (Quoted in Hill 1979, 275)

The extraordinary story of blindness reveals itself in the realm of the ordinary, and thus it is only fitting that I conclude with a return to it. Blindness is revealed in a never-ending conversation between it and sightedness. The story I end with depicts such a conversation.

It is the story of a conversation between Frederick and Rod. Rod is blind and Frederick is sighted. They meet at a bar, and their conversation soon turns to the topic of shaving. What emerges is the extraordinary character of the relation between blindness and sightedness. There is nothing difficult or sophisticated about shaving. It is a common and ordinary activity. Yet, the conversation between sightedness and blindness is mediated by the ordinary, thereby revealing the extraordinary nature of the human condition.

SHAVING

'Cheers,' she said in a voice that seemed to bring the very word alive. She set the pint of beer down on the table and said, 'There it is, and I'll take your empty.' Giving another cheerful 'Cheers,' she said, 'And here's your white wine.'

They thanked her and continued their conversation almost as though they hadn't been interrupted. It was the first time Rod had been in this bar and he quite liked it. It was late in the evening, after sunset. His sight, what was left of it, was at its best in artificial lighting. Rod had come to almost despise the sunlight in the past few months. The sight loss he had experienced over this time was incredible. He only had a little to begin with. How did the ophthalmologist put it? Oh yes, 5 per cent and now it's down to 2. He had much more difficulty getting around now. He especially hated entering a building from the bright sunshine. This removed what little sight he had left.

Dark outside and artificial light inside, Rod liked the bar. It felt good. He felt comfortable and relaxed. It was small and crowded and he liked this too. Everything seemed close, cosy. He felt in control.

'What's that, what is that?' asked Frederick, pointing his finger first to his own cheek and then to Rod's.

'What?' Rod replied.

'The thing, that thing on your face,' Frederick continued in a rapid voice. 'Hey, you cut yourself shaving.'

Rod put his fingers to his cheek and touched it lightly. 'Yeah, yeah,' he said.

'Geez, you cut yourself shaving,' repeated Frederick. 'What do you use, like a regular straight razor?'

Rod removed his fingers from his cheek and curled them around his fresh pint of beer. 'Yeah, you know, a razor. What do you use?'

'Well, a razor,' answered Frederick. He laughed and pointed to Rod's cheek once more. 'But you, you should ... I mean I can see.'

'So,' Rod said in a voice that combined both hurt and sarcasm.

Frederick continued to laugh. But it wasn't one long or even hearty laugh. Instead, it was that sort of laugh interrupted by many body movements, which themselves seem to fill the gaps of laughter with more of the same. 'So, what do you mean "so"? So I can see. So you can't.' All along Frederick leaned back and then forward, leaned slightly to one side, then to the other. In a succession of staccato movements, he moved the elbow of his right arm onto the table and off again. Curiously, at least to Rod, in the midst of all this laughter emanating from Frederick's lips and body, he continued pointing, now to his own cheek, now to Rod's. It was as though Frederick's entire being was involved in this pointing.

'Yeah, I know,' said Rod. 'But, I still have to shave.'

'Sure, sure,' said Frederick quickly. 'A straight razor? I mean, you cut yourself.'

Rod watched Frederick's finger, still pointing at their faces, through the corner of his eye. But to say this, and leave it at that, would be too much of a cliché and, for Rod, 'corner of the eye' was anything but. That's all he had, after all. Corners of his eyes were all that was left of the little vision Rod had. Whatever he could see, he saw through the corners of his eyes. Everything else, in the middle, as Rod liked to think of it, was gone, just gone.

Rod sipped his beer and put it down slowly, still letting his fingers lightly caress the pint. 'I know,' he said. 'But only sometimes. I don't always cut myself.'

Becoming more and more interested in the whole thing, Frederick said, 'No, sure, but that's not really the point. I mean, the point is that you cut yourself 'cause you're blind.'

It was Rod's turn to laugh. ''Cause I'm blind!' He echoed Frederick's words in a way that showed that either he didn't understand the issue or that he disagreed with it. It wasn't that he spoke these words in order to give both impressions. Rod really didn't know. He laughed again but, this time, more at his own confusion than at anything else. He wondered what Frederick meant. He suddenly became aware that he could no longer see

Frederick's pointing finger. Just as suddenly, he realized that Frederick's face was making an appearance out of the corner of his eye.

'It's true,' Frederick said more seriously than before. 'I mean, shaving's not part of blindness.'

'Well, what the hell is?' Rod exclaimed in a tone that oozed disgust.

In a voice that seemed to be synchronized with the movement of his hands, Frederick said, 'Yeah, yeah, that's what I mean. It's not part of blindness, so' – he drew this word out – 'why not use an electric razor?'

'I can't,' Rod replied. 'I tried it, it just gives me, well, I've got really sensitive skin and it gives me a rash. I mean, it's just crazy, it's a weird rash.'

'Really?' Frederick said.

'Yeah, that's why I never used to shave,' Rod said. 'Remember, remember, I used to have that really short beard. Remember, the Don Johnson look.'

'Right, right,' Frederick said, this time his arms folded on the table in front of him.

Frederick disappeared from the corner of Rod's eye. Rod noticed, more through hearing than anything else, some movement at the table next to them. It was quite a commotion. The people who had been sitting there were leaving, and a new group was taking their place almost before the others had left. 'Sorry,' said Rod. 'Is that in your way?' He leaned over to move his bag.

'No, no.' The reply came from somewhere in the commotion. Rod couldn't really tell from where. He looked over and smiled anyway.

Frederick followed this exchange with his eyes. He too cast a smile toward the commotion. Leaning back and forth slightly but still keeping his arms folded in front of him, Frederick said, 'But now you're shaving again.' Laughing and again doing so with both his voice and body, Frederick said, 'So, a new look.' As if someone else had said this, Frederick seemed a little surprised and even amused and began, once more, to speak with his hands. 'You know, I mean a look, a look, now that's part of blindness. It's not just for you. You know, it's like for people who can see. It's like you create a look, you know, for yourself but then the look is for the others to see. It's kind of like an orientation.'

'Of course,' Rod said, more interested now and also beginning to speak with his hands. 'It's like how you hav'ta be in the world.'

'Sure, sure,' Frederick replied. 'But still, if a blind guy is going to shave, it's like anything else, you have to use the right technology.'

Rod responded with a look. He raised his eyebrows, smiled, and nodded slightly.

Frederick must have seen the look since he replied, 'It's true. I mean, when you read, you don't read a book, I mean, a printed book. You have it, you know what I mean? You have it on tape. So you read, you read like a blind guy, you know what I mean?'

'Yeah,' Rod replied and added yet another look to his reply.

His body still animating his voice, Frederick said, 'It's the electric razor, the electric razor is technology.' Reaching out and touching Rod lightly on the arm, he said, 'It's like, it's like the electric razor, it's like that, what do you call it, that talking computer.'

'How you guys doing?' They were interrupted by the waitress. 'Ready for another?' she asked, just as cheerfully as before.

Frederick tipped the remaining wine from his glass into his mouth and said, 'Sure.'

Giving the waitress a look, Rod smiled, handed her his empty pint and said, 'Yeah, that's great.'

The waitress returned Rod's look, thinking that he could see it, and asked, 'Are you interested in a menu at all?'

Rod turned his look on Frederick. 'What do you think?' he asked. 'Are you ...?'

Looking first at Rod, then at the waitress, and finally at Rod again, Frederick said, 'Sure, sure.'

'Be right back,' she said, and was gone so quickly that her image never did linger in the corner of Rod's eye.

'Bubbly,' Rod said, smiling.

'Yeah, really. Anyway,' Frederick continued, 'so shaving is like an activity in the world and you are, you know, a blind guy, and you have to find technology. See, you know what I mean, the electric razor, that's the technology.'

'What are you saying?' asked Rod. 'You mean shaving's a visual thing? I mean shaving with a straight razor.'

'Yeah, exactly!' Frederick said, his hands speaking more loudly than ever now.

'Well, when you shave,' Rod said, his hands now in conversation with Frederick's, 'is it all sight when you shave? You know, is it just visual?'

'Exactly, exactly,' Frederick replied. 'It's visual. You just look in the mirror and you do it all by sight.'

Rod was very curious now. 'You mean you don't sort of touch, you know, feel your face?' he asked.

Frederick seemed more intrigued than curious and said, 'No, no, you just look! It's all done by sight.'

'See, 'cause what I do,' said Rod, 'well, I feel my face. I feel everything and I go over the same spot, you know, about a hundred times.'

'No wonder you cut yourself,' Frederick said, laughing.

'Yeah,' Rod continued, 'I keep feeling one spot until it's perfectly smooth. You know, I keep shaving it.'

'Well, that's wrong,' Frederick said. 'You look to see if it's smooth. Smooth is like a visual thing, not a touch thing, at least for shaving.'

Rod continued as if he were engaged in some sort of Royal Commission. 'Well, what do you do?' he asked. 'You just stand there in front of the mirror and when it looks smooth you stop?'

'Right, right,' replied Frederick, just as serious as Rod was about this inquiry.

'Well see,' Rod said, 'I use a lot of shaving cream, I mean I use a ton. I figure this helps. You know, if I use enough shaving cream, I won't cut myself.'

'No, no,' Frederick said, touching Rod lightly on the arm again. 'It's like you use very little, very little.'

'Really!'

'Yeah, hardly any. In fact, you know, I don't even use it.'

Rod's eyes opened even wider. Frederick was once again in the corner of his eyes.

'No, really,' continued Frederick. 'I don't use that stuff.'

'Well, what do you do?' asked Rod with a curiosity so genuine that it seemed to startle Frederick.

'What do you mean?'

'Well,' Rod repeated, 'what do you use? I mean if not shaving cream, what?'

'Hot water, just a little hot water.'

'Really?'

'Yeah,' said Frederick, 'just a little hot water. That's what I mean. I mean it's a visual thing. You just look and shave what you can see. Then if you can't see it ...'

'Then what?' Rod was so curious now that his body was more involved in the conversation than Frederick's.

'Well, well then, you don't shave it. I mean, you have to see. You have to look and then you can see whether or not this place or that place.' Frederick was now pointing to various spots on his face. 'You can see what places need shaving.'

A look of disappointment seemed to spread down from Rod's face to his entire body. Slightly nodding, and not smiling now, he said, 'So, just a little hot water. And then, and then, you just look and see.'

'That's right.'

There was a slight pause, and both were now leaning back in their chairs. They had that look about them which is often seen in those who have just finished something important and whose countenance now breathes a sigh of satisfaction smudged a little with disappointment. But their eyes revealed a wonder that betrayed the look of their bodies. It was as though conclusion came wrapped in the dangling sense of something yet unsaid.

The pause was interrupted by the cheerful voice. 'Here you go,' she said. 'Your beer and your white wine. Cheers!'

'Cheers,' they said almost simultaneously.

'Wait.' Turning to Rod, Frederick said, 'Do you want ... do you want? Ah, should we eat?'

The cheerful voice flooded over them once more. 'Would you like to see menus?'

'Yeah, do you?' asked Rod.

'Sure, sure. Sure, we'll see menus,' said Frederick, making the decision official.

With a quick 'Be right back,' she was gone.

Shifting in his chair and leaning forward, Rod looked at Frederick and asked, 'Where's the, ah, where's the men's room? Do you know?'

'Yeah,' replied Frederick. 'Do you want, do you want?'

'No, no, just, ah ...'

Pointing, Frederick said, 'You just go there to the end, turn right ...'

'What,' Rod interrupted, 'are you pointing?'

'Yeah, yeah sorry. You go to your right to the end, to the wall. It's just past these tables.'

'Then?'

'Then you turn, let's see, you turn right. There's a door there. Then you open it.' Frederick gave this last instruction slowly and laughed.

'Yeah, yeah,' said Rod, standing by this time. 'The door, then what?'

'Well, then you open it and there's stairs.'

'One flight?'

'I think so. Yeah one flight,' said Frederick. 'Then there's two doors on the left. I think, I think it's the last one.'

'You think? Do you know?'

'No, not exactly,' said Frederick. 'Do you want, do you want?'

'No, it's okay, I'll find it.' And, with that, Rod left the table.

Frederick sipped his wine and watched as Rod proceeded slowly to his right.

Rod made sure that he kept the tables in the corner of his eye. 'A wall,' he thought, reminding himself. He had put his right hand in his pocket but kept his left arm slightly in front of him. The fingers of this hand curled slightly in an expectant way. 'Okay, the wall, right, and now the door,' he reminded himself. Rod located the door, found the doorknob, and opened it. His eyes were immediately hit with a white so bright that it blinded him the rest of the way. 'Fuck,' he whispered to himself. 'That's bright! I'm going to have to get one of those fucking white sticks one of these days.' Rod stopped immediately in mid-step. He stood there for a few seconds. By this time, his left hand was on the door jamb. He held the door open with his right leg and slowly moved his left foot forward. His left hand, moving almost independently, was now on the wall beyond the door. Almost as though it was choreographed, his right hand began searching for a bannister.

Frederick lit one of Rod's cigarettes and continued to sip his wine. He remembered to place Rod's cigarettes and lighter back exactly where he had found them. He wondered if Rod had found the washroom alright, and then his thoughts shifted to shaving.

Keeping his feet firmly planted, Rod leaned as far forward as he dared and continued his search for a bannister. His right hand finally located one. Relieved, Rod straightened and slowly began to move forward. At about the time his left foot found the first stair, his left hand discovered, and it really was a discovery, yet another bannister. Rod thought of this discovery as a piece of good luck. Most stairways, especially in buildings this old, had only one bannister, if they had one at all. He now had both hands firmly on the bannisters and proceeded down the stairs slowly. He remembered thinking that every one of his steps was like a reconnaissance mission. He was judging the space between his steps, the depth of the stairs, whether or not the steps were uniformly spaced, and everything else that goes with walking down a flight of stairs, at least, he thought, everything that goes with him. Rod didn't have to remind himself to count the stairs since that had become a natural thing for him, especially in the last couple of years. The stairs seemed uniformly spaced and Rod counted twelve. There was no thirteenth stair, but he still hung onto the bannisters and slid his right foot forward as far as he could, just to make sure. Rod's left hand left the bannister as quickly as it had found it. His hand now on the wall beyond the stairs, Rod forged ahead, his hand searching for the first doorway.

'A visual event, that's interesting,' Frederick thought. 'A phone call,' he thought, 'probably wasn't. There's a phone call, two people having a conversation not being able to see each other. But shaving,' he mused, 'that's different. Not that Rod shouldn't shave,' thought Frederick, 'but he should use an electric razor. An electric razor wouldn't change shaving into a feeling event.' Frederick smiled at this feeling event.

Rod's hand found the door jamb. He had located the first door. The second door was not more than two feet away from the first. 'Shit,' Rod thought, 'I don't know which one of these is mine.' Just then, Rod was slightly startled by a voice. It came from the second door. 'Oh sorry,' the voice said. It was without question a male voice. Rod laughed and said, 'That's okay.' The voice then disappeared up the stairs. Rod continued to laugh to himself. He laughed because he knew he had got lucky yet again. He passed through the door that the voice had left open for him. 'Again lucky,' Rod thought. The lighting in the men's room was dull and not bright. Rod knew he would have no trouble finding the urinal.

'In one way,' thought Frederick, 'the whole world is a sighted event.' Frederick suddenly began to think how he would get along in the world if he couldn't see. Almost as suddenly, the word 'artful' sprung to his mind. He smiled, sipped his wine, and thought that perhaps blindness is really the ultimate test for artfulness.

Rod ran his hands under some warm water and, before leaving the bathroom, looked into the mirror above the sink. It occurred to him just then that the only reason he looked in the mirror while he was shaving was because it was above the sink. 'Where else could he look?' he thought. He looked in the mirror because it was there. The corner of Rod's eye caught his mirror image, and he turned to leave the men's room.

'Menus.' The cheerful voice was back. She placed one menu in front of Frederick and turned to place the other one on the table in front of Rod's empty chair.

Reaching his hand toward the menu, Frederick said, 'No, no that's okay, he's ...'

'Sorry, what?'

'He's partially sighted, you know ...'

The waitress brought the downward movement of the menu to an immediate stop as if it were about to land in something dangerous. 'He's what?'

'He can't read it,' replied Frederick. 'I mean, he can't see it. He's, like, ah, blind.'

'Really?' The waitress jerked the menu back to her side.

'Yeah,' said Frederick slowly. 'Actually, he can see a little.'

'I see.' The waitress laughed, but, this time, it didn't seem quite as cheerful. 'Back in a minute,' she said and retreated from the table.

'Partially sighted. Geez,' Frederick thought, 'what the hell does that mean?' He felt a little silly and continued sipping his wine.

Returning to the table was fairly easy, which is to say fairly routine, for Rod. After all, falling up stairs was certainly less dangerous than falling down them. Moreover, he had those bannisters; Rod loved bannisters. Through the door and out of the blinding light, Rod paused for a moment. He regained himself and slowly made his way back to the table.

'Hey, you made it,' Frederick said in a somewhat mocking tone.

Rod felt the back of the chair and, sliding his hand down the chair's arm, sat.

'Did you find it okay?' asked Frederick.

'Yeah,' replied Rod confidently. 'It was the second door just like you said. No problem.'

'She brought menus.'

'Oh great.'

'Geez, I told her, I told her you were partially sighted,' said Frederick.

'What?'

'You know, she brought the menus. She brought two. So I said, I said he can't read it, he's partially sighted.'

'So, what did she do?' asked Rod.

'She just took it away,' replied Frederick.

'Oh yeah.'

'Yeah,' continued Frederick, 'but she was a little surprised. Geez, I mean, you should have a white ... thing, you know, white cane.'

'Why,' asked Rod rhetorically, 'just for her, just to make her feel better?'

'Well, kind of,' said Frederick thoughtfully. 'I mean, no one knows. She thinks ... the guy can't read. What do ya' mean partially sighted?'

'Yeah,' now thoughtful himself, Rod said. 'I know what you mean. I'm going to have to start using a white cane one of these days.'

'Don't look so gloomy,' Frederick said laughing. 'It's better than saying you're partially sighted.'

'You think?' asked Rod, returning his fingers to his cheek once more.

'Yeah,' Frederick replied. 'It doesn't mean anything. You know, you say partially sighted, but there's no content. No one knows.'

'I know,' said Rod. 'It's like telling someone you only have part of what they have. Then, you figure, you figure they'd say "What part?"'

'Yeah,' Frederick said slowly. 'It's like trying to get a sense of a part. I have everything, you have some. I mean, it makes no sense.'

Touching his cheek, Rod said, 'It's true, it's true. I mean, I tell people I'm partially sighted when I'm trying to explain something. You know, I tell them when I'm trying to find something in a store, or something like that. But, you know, I don't think it's the partial thing that's confusing. I think it's the sighted thing.'

'What about partially blind?' asked Frederick. 'Tell them that.'

'I should try,' said Rod laughing. 'It's like partially blind means almost blind. So, partially sighted ...'

'Yeah,' interrupted Frederick. 'Partially blind means that. It's like the word *blind,* I mean I tell someone that you can hardly see.'

'I guess partially sighted means you can almost see,' laughed Rod. 'I guess, then, they don't know what to do, who would?'

She was back and, this time, more cheerful than ever, or at least it seemed this way to Rod. 'Did you have a chance to take a look? ... I mean, have you ...?' The waitress laughed and looked at Frederick. She wondered if her face was red and chided herself for what she thought was an excessive laugh. She felt the discomfort overcome her and knew she should say something to break this silence. Relief invaded her discomfort as she heard Rod speak.

'This guy hasn't read a thing to me,' laughed Rod. 'I'm not sure he can see either.'

She turned to Rod and her cheerfulness betrayed her relief. Putting her hand on Rod's shoulder, she said, 'Can't trust anyone nowadays.' Rod smiled and she relaxed back into her cheerfulness. She offered to tell Rod what the specials were, and when she laughed this time, she did not feel it to be excessive. Comfortable once more, she left with their orders.

Rod knew that he had made the waitress feel more comfortable. But more important than this, he knew that it was he who caused her to be uncomfortable in the first place. This made him uncomfortable.

'My turn,' said Frederick, interrupting Rod's thoughts.

'Second door on your left,' said Rod.

Frederick laughed and left Rod with his discomfort.

Rod waited. He began to fight his discomfort. 'Why shouldn't the waitress feel uncomfortable?' he thought. Shit, he did. He wondered if a white cane would make him feel more comfortable with himself or, for that matter, whether or not it would make others feel more comfortable. It would certainly let people know that he was blind or, he smiled, that he was partially blind. Rod wondered what being comfortable with blindness would feel like. What it would look like? Could blindness be comforting? he wondered. The expression 'comfort zone' suddenly sprung to his

mind. He chuckled as he remembered the yuppies, or so he characterized them, who use this phrase and the cavalier way in which they do. Rod
laughed again and thought that being in a zone would be the only way to
be comfortable with blindness.

Dismissing these thoughts as themselves cavalier, he returned his mind
to the waitress. He had made her feel more comfortable, and something
about this made him uncomfortable. He wondered how that worked. He
didn't like making people feel that way.

'Hey, hey,' Frederick said in a way that served to announce his return.
'You're right, it was the second door.'

'Bright down there,' Rod said.

'Really?'

Cheerful and feeling comfortable, the waitress served the pair their
meals. While they ate, they discussed some research project with which
Frederick was involved. Blindness was not mentioned for the rest of the
evening, and both of them left the bar wondering whether or not this was
intentional.

Rod arrived at his apartment door, felt for the key hole, and inserted
his key. He entered and pressed the button on his watch. The computer
voice told him that it wasn't too late, only eleven-o-one-P-M. 'Good,' he
thought, and proceeded to his bathroom.

Rod stood at the sink and looked at himself in the mirror. His hand
moved slowly upwards, and the corner of his eye saw his fingers gently
caressing the small cut on his cheek.

Bibliography

Arendt, Hannah. 1958. *The Human Condition*. Chicago: University of Chicago Press
- 1968. *Men in Dark Times*. New York: Harcourt Brace Jovanovich
- 1971. *Life of the Mind*. New York: Harcourt Brace Jovanovich
- 1982. *Lectures on Kant's Political Philosophy*. Chicago: University of Chicago Press
- 1994. *Essays in Understanding 1930–1954*. New York: Harcourt Brace
Aristotle. 1962. *Nichomachean Ethics*. Indianapolis: Liberal Arts Press
Barraga, Natalie. 1983. *Visual Handicaps and Learning*. Austin, Texas: Exceptional Resources
Bataille, Georges. 1985. *Visions of Excess: Selected Writings, 1927–1939*. Trans. Allan Stoekl. Minneapolis: University of Minnesota Press
Baudrillard, Jean. 1987. *The Ecstasy of Communication*. Trans. Bernard and Caroline Schutze. New York: Semiotext(e)
Beckett, Samuel. 1954. *Waiting for Godot: A Tragicomedy in Two Acts*. New York: Grove Press
Berger, John. 1972. *Ways of Seeing*. London: British Broadcasting Corporation
Berger, Peter. 1963. *Invitation to Sociology: A Humanistic Perspective*. New York: Doubleday
Blum, Alan. 1982. 'Victim, Patient, Client, Pariah: Steps in the Self-Understanding of the Experience of Suffering and Affliction.' *Reflections: Canadian Journal of Visual Impairment* 1: 64–82
Blum, Alan, and Peter McHugh. 1984. *Self Reflection in the Arts and Sciences*. Atlantic Highlands, N.J.: Humanities Press
Bonner, Kieran. 1984. 'The Social Construction of Birth Announcements.' Paper presented at the Canadian Learned Society, Guelph, Ont.
- 1997. *A Great Place to Raise Kids: Interpretation, Science, and the Urban-Rural Debate*. Montreal and Kingston: McGill-Queen's University Press

Cholden, Louis S. 1958. *A Psychiatrist Works with Blindness.* New York: American
    Foundation for the Blind
Cicero. 1971. *On the Good Life.* Trans. Michael Grant. New York: Penguin Books
Classen, Constance. 1993. *World of Sense: Exploring the Senses in History and across
    Cultures.* New York: Routledge
Derrida, Jacques. 1978. *Writing and Difference.* Trans. Alan Bass. Chicago: Univer-
    sity of Chicago Press
- 1993. *Memoirs of the Blind: The Self-Portrait and Other Ruins.* Trans. Pascale-Anne
    Brault and Michael Naas. Chicago: University of Chicago Press
Descartes, Rene. 1993. *Discourse on Method and Meditations on First Philosophy.* Trans.
    D.A. Cress. 3rd ed. Indianapolis: Hackett Publishing Company
Diderot, Denis. 1982. 'Diderot's Letter on the Blind for the Use of Those Who
    See.' *Reflections: Canadian Journal of Visual Impairment* 1: 83–122
Durkheim, Emile. 1938. *The Rules of Sociological Method.* New York: Free Press
Erikson, E.H. 1968. *Identity, Youth and Crisis.* New York: W.W. Norton
Foucault, Michel. 1973. *The Birth of the Clinic: An Archaeology of Medical Perception.*
    New York: Tavistock
Fraiberg, Selma. 1977. *Insights from the Blind: Studies of Blind and Sighted Infants.*
    New York: Basic Books
Frankl, Victor E. 1962. *Man's Search for Meaning: An Introduction to Logotherapy.*
    Boston: Beacon Press
- 1969. *The Will to Meaning: Foundations and Applications of Logotherapy.* New York:
    World Publishing Company
Gadacz, Rene R., ed. 1994. *Rethinking Disability: New Structures, New Relationships.*
    Edmonton: University of Alberta Press
Gadamer, Hans-Georg. 1975. *Truth and Method.* New York: Crossroad Publishing
    Company
- 1996. *The Enigma of Health: The Art of Healing in a Scientific Age.* Trans. Jason
    Gaiger and Nicholas Walker. Stanford: Stanford University Press
Garfinkel, Harold. 1967. *Studies in Ethnomethodology.* Englewood Cliffs, N.J.:
    Prentice-Hall
Goffman, Erving. 1959. *The Presentation of Self in Everyday Life.* New York: Double-
    day Anchor Books
- 1963. *Stigma: Notes on the Management of Spoiled Identity.* Englewood Cliffs, N.J.:
    Prentice-Hall
Gombrich, E.H. 1960. *Art and Illusion: A Study in the Psychology of Pictorial Representa-
    tion.* Princeton: Princeton University Press
Gott, Ted (compiler). 1994. *Don't Leave Me This Way: Art in the Age of AIDS.*
    Victoria: National Gallery of Australia

Hacking, Ian. 1986. 'Making Up People.' In *Individuality and the Self in Western Thought.* Ed. A. Heller, S. Sosna, and L. Wellbery. Stanford: Stanford University Press. 102–31

Harrison, Felicity, and Mary Crow. 1993. *Living and Learning with Blind Children: A Guide for Parents and Teachers of Visually Impaired Children.* Toronto: University of Toronto Press

Heidegger, Martin. 1966. *Discourse on Thinking.* Trans. John M. Anderson and E. Hans Freund. New York: Harper Torchbooks

– 1968. *What Is Called Thinking.* Trans. J. Glen Gray. New York: Harper Colophon Books

– 1977. *The Question Concerning Technology: And Other Essays.* Trans. William Lovitt. New York: Harper and Row

Higgins, Paul. 1992. *Making Disability: Exploring the Social Transformation of Human Variation.* Springfield, Ill.: Charles C. Thomas, Publishers

Hill, Melvyn A. 1979. 'The Fictions of Mankind and the Stories of Men.' In *Hannah Arendt: The Recovery of the Public World.* Ed. Melvyn A. Hill. New York: St Martin's Press. 275–300

Hillyer, Barbara. 1993. *Feminism and Disability.* Norman, Okla.: University of Oklahoma Press

Hippocrates. 1978. *Hippocratic Writings.* Trans. J. Chadwick and N.N. Mann. New York: Penguin Books

Homer. 1979. *The Iliad.* Trans. E.V. Rieu. New York: Penguin Books

– 1980. *The Odyssey.* Trans. E.V. Rieu. New York: Penguin Books

Howes, David, ed. 1991. *The Varieties of Sensory Experience: A Source Book in the Anthropology of the Senses.* Toronto: University of Toronto Press

Jay, Martin. 1994. *Downcast Eyes: The Denigration of Vision in Twentieth-Century French Thought.* Berkeley: University of California Press

Jenks, Chris, ed. 1995. *Visual Culture.* London: Routledge

Karatheodoris, Stephen. 1982. 'Blindness, Illusion and the Need for an Image of Sight.' *Reflections: Canadian Journal of Visual Impairment* 1: 31–51

Kidel, Mark. 1988. 'Illness and Meaning.' In *The Meaning of Illness.* Ed. M. Kidel and S. Rowe-Lete. New York: Routledge. 3–36

Kierkegaard, Søren. 1941a. *Concluding Unscientific Postscript.* Trans. David F. Swenson and Walter Lowrie. Princeton: Princeton University Press

– 1941b. *Fear and Trembling and the Sickness unto Death.* Trans. W. Lowrie. Princeton: Princeton University Press

Kosinski, Jerzy. 1970. *Being There.* Toronto: Bantam Books

Kunc, Norman. 1981. *Ready, Willing and Disabled.* Toronto: Personal Library

Kushner, Harold S. 1981. *When Bad Things Happen to Good People.* New York: Avon Books

Lacan, Jacques. 1977. *Ecrits: A Selection.* Trans. Alan Sheridan. New York: W.W. Norton

Leder, Drew. 1990. *The Absent Body.* Chicago: University of Chicago Press

Levin, David M. 1988. *The Opening of Vision: Nihilism and the Postmodern Situation.* New York: Routledge

– ed. 1993. *Modernity and the Hegemony of Vision.* Berkeley: University of California Press

Levine, Les. 1976. *I Am Not Blind: An Information Environment about Unsighted People.* Hartford: Wadsworth Athenaeum

Littlejohn, Stephen. 1989. *Theories of Human Communication.* Belmont, Calif.: Wadsworth

McHugh, Peter. 1993. 'Making, Fragmentation, and the End of Endurance.' *Dianoia: A Liberal Arts Interdisciplinary Journal* 3(1): 41–51

– 1994. 'Insomnia and the (T)error of Postmodernism.' Paper presented to the Society for Phenomenology and the Social Sciences, Seattle

McHugh, Peter, et al. 1974. *On the Beginning of Social Inquiry.* London: Routledge and Kegan Paul

Merleau-Ponty, M. 1962. *Phenomenology of Perception.* Trans. Colin Smith. London: Routledge and Kegan Paul

– 1964. *The Primacy of Perception: And Other Essays on Phenomenological Psychology, the Philosophy of Art, History and Politics.* Evanston, Ill.: Northwestern University Press

– 1968. *The Visible and the Invisible.* Evanston, Ill.: Northwestern University Press

Michalko, Rod. 1978. 'Reading Aloud.' Unpublished paper

– 1982. 'Passing: Accomplishing the Sighted World.' *Reflections: Canadian Journal of Visual Impairment* 1: 9–30

– 1984. 'The Metaphor of Adolescence.' *Phenomenology and Pedagogy: A Human Science Journal* 1(3): 296–311

– 1987. 'The Birth of Disability.' *Phenomenology and Pedagogy* 5(2): 119–31

– 1988. 'Natural Childbirth, Physical Fitness and Natural Foods: The Purification of the Body under Modern Conditions.' Paper presented to the Society for Phenomenology and the Human Sciences, Toronto

– 1990. 'Ethnography and Childhood Blindness.' In *Through the Looking Glass: Children and Health Promotion.* Ottawa: Canadian Public Health Association. 175–82

– 1996a. 'White as a Cane: Stories of Blindness.' Unpublished manuscript

– 1996b. 'The Opening of the Bureaucratic Mind: Putting Good Works into Practice.' Paper presented at the CIRLA conference, Banff, Alberta

Parisian, Doug. 1981. 'Education and Afterward.' In *The Positive Path: Profiles of Disabled Manitobans*. N.p.: The Council for Exceptional Children

Piaget, Jean. 1932. *The Moral Judgement of the Child*. London: Routledge, Kegan and Paul

Plato. 1954. *The Last Days of Socrates*. New York: Penguin Books

– 1961. *The Collected Dialogues of Plato*. Ed. Edith Hamilton. Princeton: Princeton University Press

Sacks, Oliver. 1995. *An Anthropologist on Mars: Seven Paradoxical Tales*. Toronto: Alfred A. Knopf Canada

Sartre, Jean-Paul. 1948. *Anti-Semite and Jew*. Trans. George J. Becker. New York: Schocken Books

– 1956. *Being and Nothingness*. New York: Washington Square Press

– 1966. *The Psychology of Imagination*. New York: Citadel Press

Scholl, G.T., and I.J. Holman. 1981. 'Impacts of Mainstreaming during Career Building, Ages 13–21.' In *Blindness Annual 1980–81*. Washington, D.C.: American Association of Workers for the Blind. 68–82

Schutz, Alfred. 1973. *Collected Papers I: The Problem of Social Reality*. The Hague: Martinus Nijhoff

Scott, Robert. 1969. *The Making of Blind Men: A Study of Adult Socialization*. New Brunswick, N.J.: Transaction, Inc.

Shapiro, Joseph P. 1993. *No Pity: People with Disabilities Forging a New Civil Rights Movement*. New York: Random House

Smith, Dorothy. 1987. *The Everyday World as Problematic: A Feminist Sociology*. Toronto: University of Toronto Press

Sudnow, David. 1972. 'Temporal Parameters of Interpersonal Observation.' In *Studies in Social Interaction*. Ed. David Sudnow. New York: Free Press. 259–79

Synnott, Anthony. 1993. *The Body Social: Symbolism, Self and Society*. New York: Routledge

Taussig, Michael. 1993. *Memesis and Alterity: A Particular History of the Senses*. New York: Routledge

Temkin, Owsei. 1991. *Hippocrates in a World of Pagans and Christians*. Baltimore: Johns Hopkins University Press

Tolstoy, Leo. 1978. 'The Death of Ivan Ilyich.' In *'The Cossacks' and Other Stories*. New York: Penguin Books. 99–162

Tucker, Bonnie P. 1995. *The Feel of Silence*. Philadelphia: Temple University Press

Turner, Roy. 1970. 'Words, Utterances and Activities.' In *Understanding Everyday Life*. Ed. Jack D. Douglas. Chicago: Aldine. 169–87

– ed. 1974. *Ethnomethodology: Selected Readings*. Baltimore: Penguin Books

van Manen, Max. 1990. *Researching Lived Experience: Human Science for an Action Sensitive Pedagogy*. London, Ont.: Althouse Press

Weiner, Bluma, and James Gallagher. 1986. *Alternative Futures in Special Education*. Reston, Va.: Council for Exceptional Children

Wells, H.G. 1911. '*The Country of the Blind' and Other Stories*. London: T. Nelson

– 1927. *Selected Short Stories*. Harmondsworth, England: Penguin Books

Wittgenstein, Ludwig. 1958. *Philosophical Investigations*. Trans. G.E.M. Anscombe. Guildford, England: Basil Blackwell and Mott, Ltd

Zola, Irving K. 1982. *Missing Pieces: A Chronical of Living with a Disability*. Philadelphia: Temple University Press

Index

accessibility, 40–7, 89, 95, 147

accommodation: coping practices, 28–9; 'fitting in,' 132–3. *See also techné*

adolescence: and convention, 101; 'fundamental anxiety' of, 109, 114–15; as a relation, 96–7, 99–102, 123, 125–6, 138

adulthood. *See* maturity

Arendt, Hannah, 83nn7, 8, 155n8, 158; 'human condition,' 109, 134; identity, 33, 33n4; understanding, 34

Aristotle: the good, 61

Bataille, Georges, 91n10

Baudrillard, Jean, 102

Beckett, Samuel, 56

Berger, Peter, 83

blindness: and adversity, 26–7, 133; collective representation of, 45–6, 110, 132, 138–9n2; as a country, 23–4; and death, 10, 30–2; as disruption, 27, 53, 92; and 'dramatic immersion,' 8; as essential incompleteness, 123; and imagination, 84–7, 145, 154; as incurable, 54–7, 64; and lack/loss, 24–6, 42, 45–6, 64, 69, 72, 74, 122, 124, 141; and making a place, 140–1; as a medical condition, 35; moral character of, 25–6; as problem/trouble, 24–7, 29, 37, 100; as a question, 154; as shadow of sight, 67–8, 77; as a social construct, 71–2, 102; as a spectacle, 47; as a teacher, 127, 133–5, 156; and technology, 28–9; vocabulary of, 71–3

blindness and sightedness: conversation of, 5, 159; mixed nature, 131; as a relation, 11, 123, 132, 149, 153; as worlds, 10

blindness prevention programs, 26, 123, 132

Blum, Alan, 30n3

Bonner, Kieran, 38, 71n1

Cholden, Louis S., 59, 61

Cicero, 141–2, 144–51, 154

Classen, Constance, 81n6

competence, 144–6

'Country of the Blind.' *See* Wells, H.G.

depiction, 148–56; versus description, 150

Derrida, Jacques, 154n7

diagnosis, 5, 35–6, 43–4, 51–9; and qualification, 37